Dental Radiology

Dental Assisting Manuals

This manual and study guide is one of a series of eight similar publications prepared to present the fundamental knowledge and skills of dental assisting.

Manual I
Professionalism, Legal Considerations, and Office Management
Ethel Earl, B.S., C.D.A.

Manual II
Basic Sciences
E. Jeff Burkes, Jr., B.S., D.D.S., M.S.
Matthew T. Wood, A.B., D.D.S., M.S.

Manual III
Preclinical Sciences
Matthew T. Wood, A.B., D.D.S., M.S.
E. Jeff Burkes, Jr., B.S., D.D.S., M.S.

Manual IV
Communication, Psychology, Nutrition, and Preventive Dentistry
Mary C. George, C.D.A., R.D.H., B.S., Ed.M.
Eleanor A. Forbes, B.S., R.D.H.
Clifton E. Crandell, B.S., D.D.S., M.S., M.Ed.

Manual V
Dental Radiology
Stephen R. Matteson, D.D.S.
Cy Whaley, B.A., R.T., Ed.D.
Vickye C. Secrist, R.D.H., B.S.

Manual VI
Dental Materials and Technical Application
Karl F. Leinfelder, D.D.S., M.S.
Roger E. Barton, D.D.S.
Duane F. Taylor, B.S.E., M.S.E., Ph.D.

Manual VII
Clinical Sciences
William D. Strickland, B.S., D.D.S.
Aldridge D. Wilder, Jr., B.S., D.D.S.

Manual VIII
Clinical Chairside Assisting
William D. Strickland, B.S., D.D.S.
Aldridge D. Wilder, Jr., B.S., D.D.S.

Dental Radiology

Fourth Edition

by Stephen R. Matteson,
Cy Whaley, and
Vickye C. Secrist

Manual V

The University of North Carolina Press
Chapel Hill

©1966, 1971, 1980, 1988 The University of North Carolina Press

Manufactured in the United States of America

96   95   6   5   4   3

Dental assisting manuals.
     Rev. ed. of: Dental assisting manual. 3rd ed. 1980.
     Includes bibliographies and index.
     Contents: v. 5 Dental radiology / Stephen R. Matteson,
Cy Whaley, and Vickye C. Secrist.
     1. Dental assistants—Handbooks, manuals, etc. 2. Dentistry
—Handbooks, manuals, etc. I. Dental assisting manual.
[DNLM: 1. Dental Assistants—handbooks. WU 39 D414]
RK60.5.D425   1988   617.6   87-16258
ISBN 0-8078-4205-2 (manual 5: pbk.)

Contents

Introduction

Dental radiographs are an extremely important aspect of dental practices in that they provide one of the most reliable diagnostic means available to the dentist. Although the amount of radiation used in dental practice is small, and the hazard to employees and patients appears to be minimal, diagnostic radiation is under close scrutiny from professional, federal, and state authorities. Thus equipment must meet certain standards, dental radiographers must meet certain minimum requirements in many states, and radiation exposure must be minimized by the use of proper techniques. Ironically, most measures prescribed to reduce radiation exposure to patients also increase the quality of the resulting radiograph. It is necessary, therefore, for all persons taking radiographs in dental offices, whether they are dentists, dental hygienists, dental assistants, or specially trained radiographers, to be adequately educated and experienced in dental radiography. Regardless of the position that the person taking dental radiographs holds in the office, the skill and knowledge concerning dental radiology must be the same and of the highest quality.

The material contained in this manual includes techniques for taking periapical films and other technical procedures, plus radiation physics, radiation biology, radiation protection, and a review of normal anatomy as identified on dental films. The revised fourth edition provides updated information on radiation safety, new and improved intraoral radiographic techniques, and additional technical information. The extensive use of illustrations throughout the manual adds significantly to the clarity of the material.

At the beginning of each section is a list of objectives for the particular section. These should be considered carefully when progressing through the material. In addition, at the end of each section is a series of questions relating to the information presented in the section. These examinations are for self-review or can be used as tests for evaluation by local instructors. They are *not* to be sent to the manual authors or publisher for grading.

The original development of the manuals was accomplished in conjunction with the preparation of an independent study program for dental assistants, sponsored through a grant from the W. K. Kellogg Foundation of Battle Creek, Michigan. The present eight manual publications are the basic information source for a series of thirty individual continuing education independent study courses for dental assistants and other dental auxiliaries conducted through Independent Study by Extension, University of North Carolina at Chapel Hill.

Many individuals, including the authors, the University of North Carolina Dental School administrators, the staff of the Learning Resources Center of the School of Dentistry, and the director and staff of the University of North Carolina Press have contributed in many ways to the revisions of these manuals. The authors sincerely appreciate the modeling services of Nancy Atwater for the preparation of the clinical photographs.

The authors of this dental radiology manual are Stephen R. Matteson, Cy Whaley, and Vickye C. Secrist. Dr. Matteson is professor and head of the Section of Oral Radiology of the Oral Diagnosis Department of the University of North Carolina School of Dentistry. Dr. Whaley is director of Allied Health and Dental Education of the Greensboro, North Carolina, Area Health Education Center. Mrs. Secrist is a clinical dental hygiene instructor and part-time supervisor at the Radiology Clinic of the University of North Carolina School of Dentistry. The editor is professor emeritus of the Ecology Department of the University of North Carolina School of Dentistry.

Roger E. Barton, Editor

Dental Radiology

Dental Radiology Practice and Equipment

Dental radiology is the clinical discipline encompassing the techniques for taking dental radiographs and the interpretation of the films to aid in obtaining a diagnosis. This section explains the role of the dental radiographer in this process and describes the x-ray equipment used.

OBJECTIVES

1. To describe and explain the formation of radiopaque and radiolucent images on a radiograph.
2. To describe the radiographic appearance of caries, periapical and periodontal disease.
3. To discuss the importance of the dental radiographer's knowledge and skills in radiology.
4. To discuss the functional parts of the Crookes tube.
5. To list three properties of cathode rays.
6. To list three properties of electromagnetic waves.
7. To list three properties of x rays.
8. To draw a diagram of the x-ray tube and label the important parts.
9. To discuss the mechanism of x-ray generation.
10. To list the components of the x-ray machine and explain their functions.
11. To list the steps to be performed when establishing the x-ray machine settings.

RADIOLOGY IN THE PRACTICE OF DENTISTRY

When a patient comes to the dental office for treatment, the dentist examines the oral cavity and decides if x rays are needed to complete a diagnosis and plan of treatment. When a new patient is examined by the dentist, a radiographic examination is usually required to complete the diagnosis because radiographs reveal hidden abnormalities that cannot be found using the clinical examination alone. The plan of treatment is determined using information obtained from both the clinical and radiographic examinations. When a recall patient is seen, x rays may be indicated to complete that examination. The dentist decides whether films are needed based on the needs of the individual patient. This decision is based upon the patient's dental history, including caries, periodontal disease, development of the dentition, and evidence of new disease clinically.

A dental radiograph is a film of the patient's teeth and jaws that is made by directing an x-ray beam through the jaw of the patient onto dental film. After the film is developed, an image of the anatomic structures can be seen and examined. Radiographs are indispensable for diagnosis because the internal structures of the teeth and jaws can be seen, and changes from normal can indicate that abnormalities are present. X rays have the unique ability to pass through materials and biologic tissues. Images of the teeth and jaws are made on the film because the x rays pass through some materials more easily than through others. Metal substances such as amalgam restorations or orthodontic wires stop all of the x rays that hit them, and because none of those rays reach the film, the film remains clear. This type of shadow on the film is called *radiopaque* because the object it represents does not allow the x-ray beam to pass through, or is opaque to the rays. Substances that are much less dense than metal, such as muscle, blood, or other soft tissues, do not stop the passage of x rays, and when radiographed, they result in blackened areas on the film. Blacker images on the film are called *radiolucent* because the radiographed object allows the x rays to pass through, or is lucent to the rays. A dental radiograph consists of an image showing many black, white, and gray shadows resulting from the variety of materials present in the mouth (Fig. 1, V-1).

Dental radiographs are used by the dentist to find many diseases. The most common dental conditions seen are dental caries, periodontal and periapical disease. These conditions destroy a portion of the normal tooth or jaw structure and therefore result in a more radiolucent shadow than is expected. Caries is a disease process that results in the destruction of tooth structure. The radiographic picture of caries is shown in Figure 2, V-1. Periodontal disease causes destruction in the soft tissues and supporting bone structure surrounding the tooth root and is illustrated in Figure 3, V-1. Periapical disease destroys alveolar bone around the apex of the tooth and is shown in Figure 4, V-1.

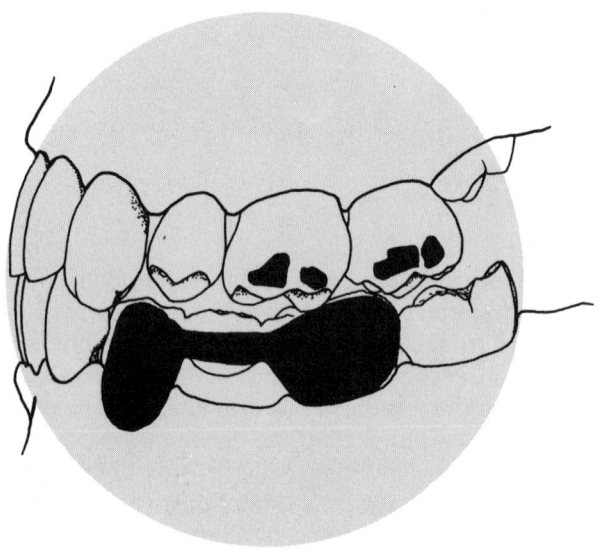

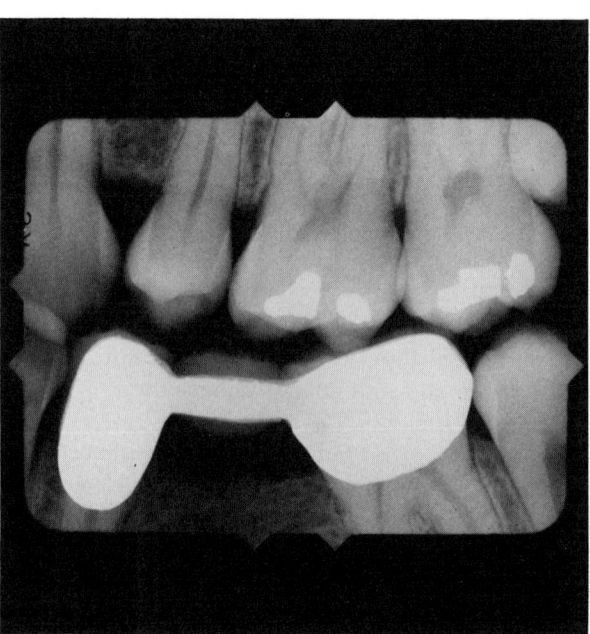

Fig. 1, V-1 Formation of the radiographic image.

A. Maxillary and mandibular left quadrants showing missing tooth no. 20, a fixed metallic bridge in place extending from tooth no. 19 to tooth no. 21, and small metallic restorations present in the maxillary molars. Area exposed with x rays when bitewing radiograph is taken (see shaded circle).

B. Resultant radiograph. X-ray beam is absorbed by metal and the film remains clear or radiopaque. The teeth absorb a large portion of the x-ray beam and are seen as various shades of gray. Radiolucent shadows represent structures through which the x rays readily penetrate, such as soft tissues.

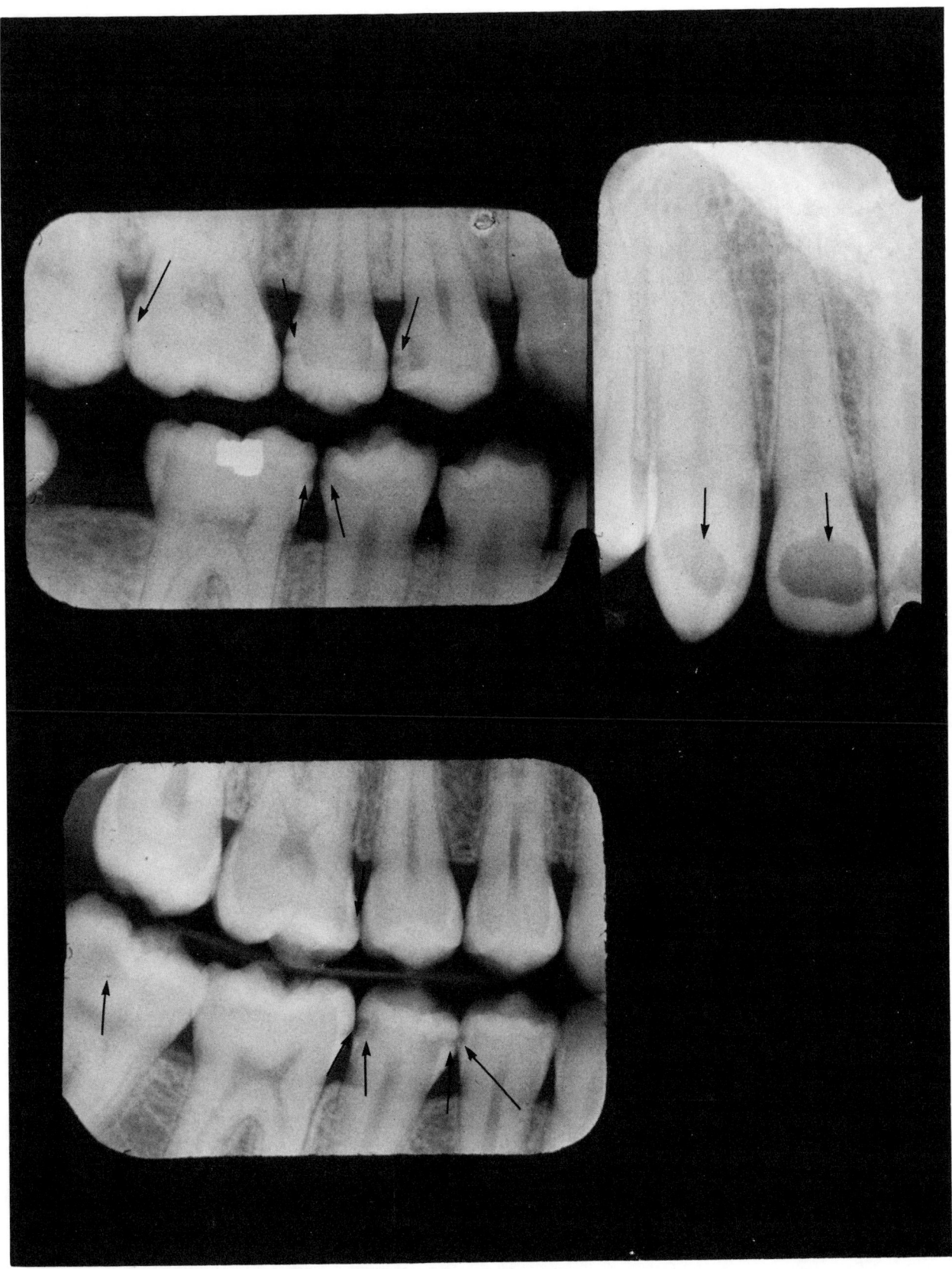

Fig. 2, V-1 Caries. Arrow denotes the radiolucent areas indicating caries.

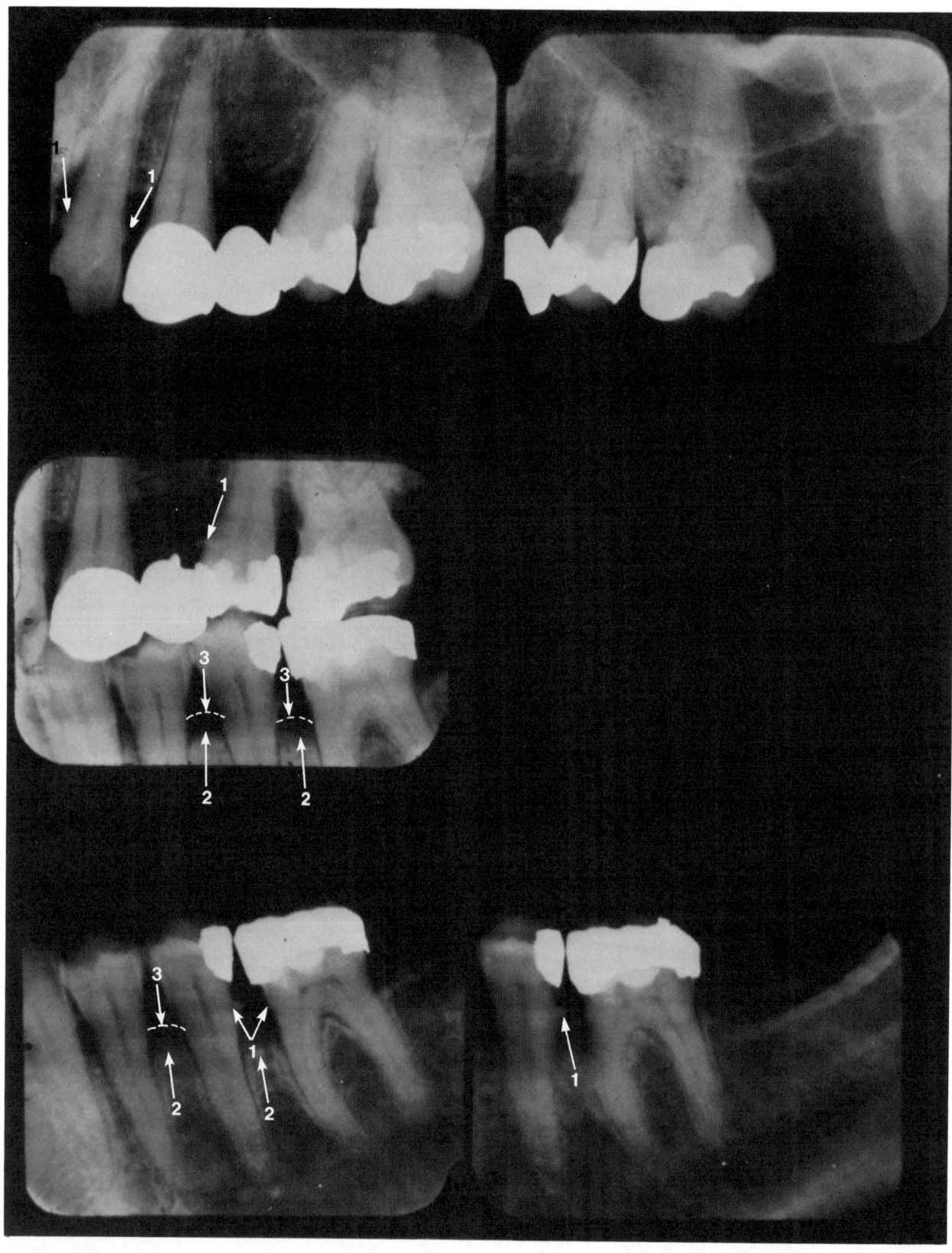

Fig. 3, V-1 Periodontal disease. (1) Calculus, (2) loss of alveolar crestal bone, (3) normal level of the bone.

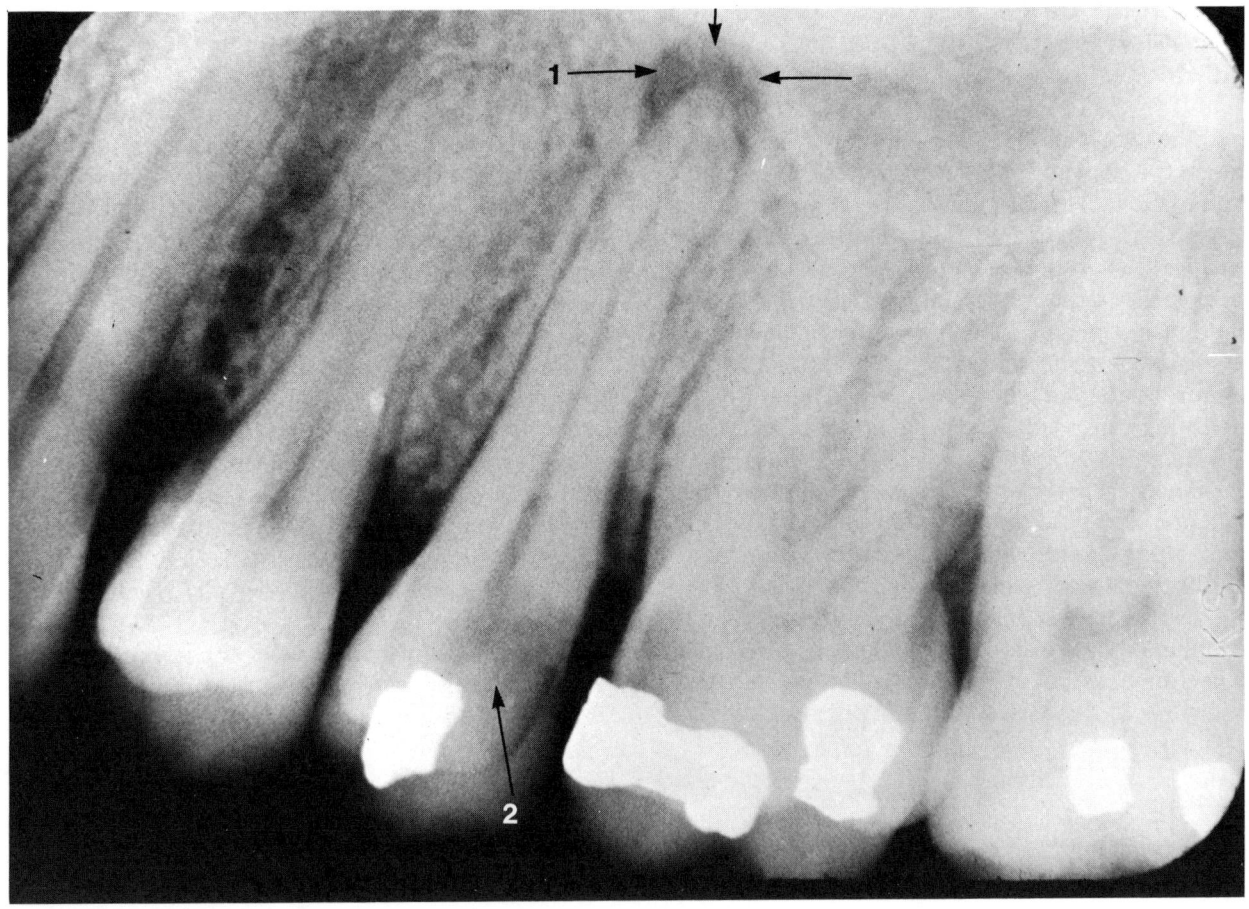

Fig. 4, V-1 Periapical disease. (1) Periapical radiolucency, (2) deep caries causing the infection.

IMPORTANCE OF THE DENTAL RADIOGRAPHER'S KNOWLEDGE AND TECHNICAL SKILLS

The dental radiographer has the very important role in the dental office of performing radiographic examinations. A well-trained and motivated dental auxiliary is valuable to both dentist and patient because this employee can be relied upon to take high-quality radiographs and to process and mount the films properly. The dentist must be able to rely on the radiographer to complete these tasks correctly because errors in radiographic technique or film mounting can result in serious errors in diagnosis and treatment.

Another important responsibility of the dental radiographer is the safe use of the x-ray equipment. Proper procedures must be used to obtain radiographs of patients while exposing the patient to the smallest practical dose of radiation. Also, radiographers should expose the radiographs using safety techniques that result in the lowest radiation exposures to themselves that are practical.

HISTORY OF RADIOLOGY

X rays were discovered by Wilhelm Conrad Roentgen in November 1895. Roentgen was a scientist who did experiments using a cathode ray tube (Crookes tube, Fig. 5, V-1). A vacuum was developed in the glass case by pumping air out of the glass case, and an electrical circuit was connected to the ends of the tube. Cathode rays, which were later shown to be streams of electrons, were seen as streams of colored light passing from the *cathode* (electrically negative) end of the tube toward the *anode* (electrically positive) end of the tube. In order to study the properties of the cathode rays, Roentgen placed an aluminum window on the side of the glass tube, permitting the cathode stream to go out into the air outside the cathode tube. He learned that cathode rays have the following characteristics:

1. Cathode rays are electrically negative particles.

2. Cathode rays can travel only a few centimeters in the air outside the cathode ray tube.

3. Cathode rays can cause a fluorescent screen

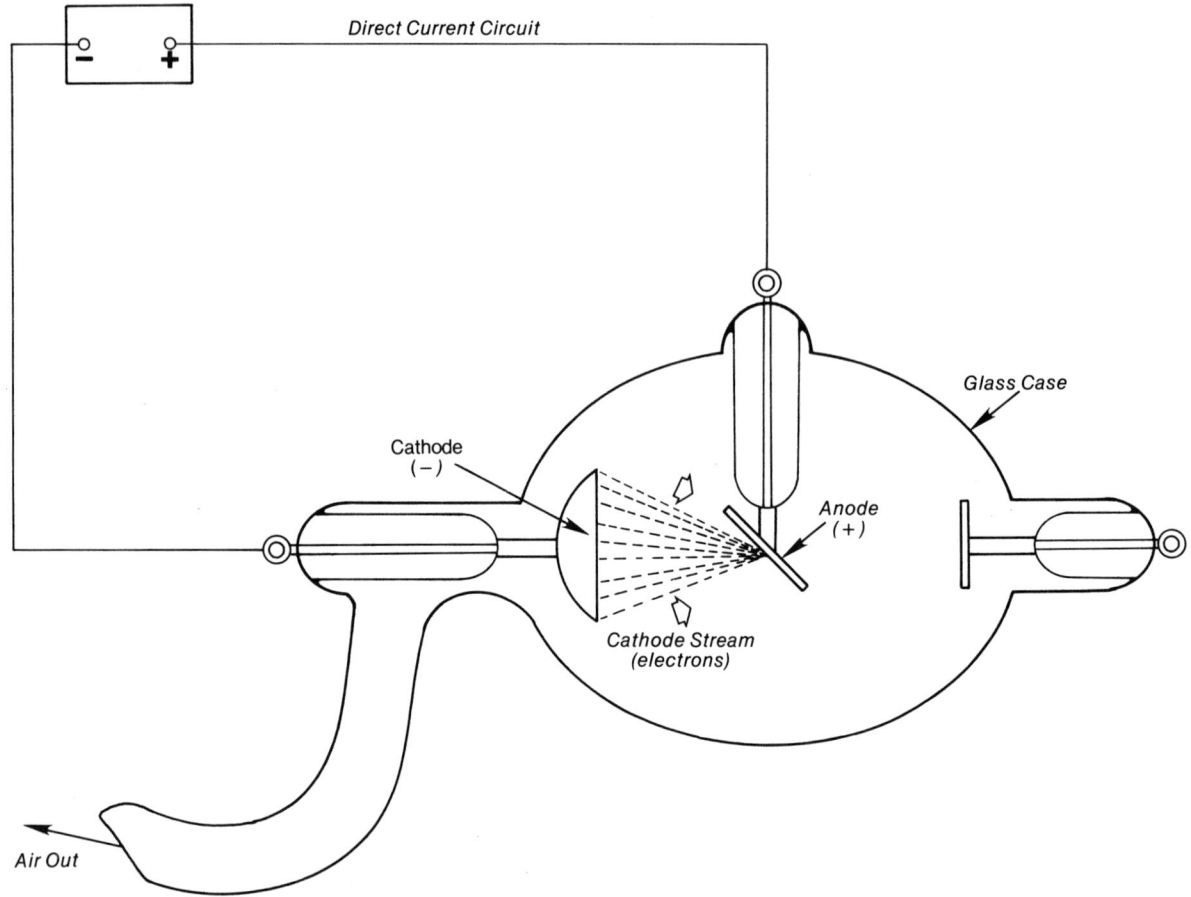

Fig. 5, V-1 Crookes tube. Cathode stream (electrons) flowing from cathode to anode.

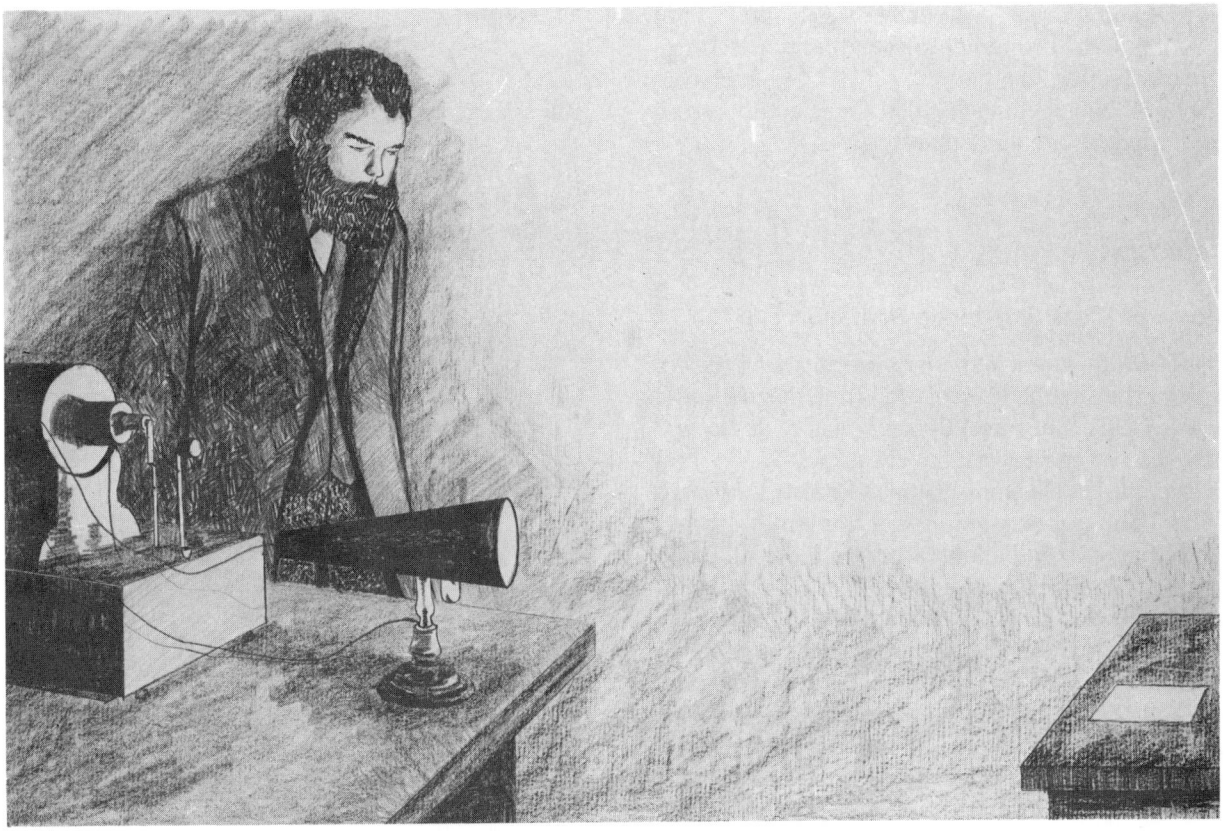

Fig. 6, V-1 Discovery of x rays. Dr. Roentgen in laboratory with Crookes tube coated with black paper. Six feet across the room, a fluorescent screen was illuminated by x rays.

to glow. A fluorescent substance will glow when struck by either light, a cathode ray beam, or an x-ray beam. An example of fluorescence is the glow of materials used on watch dials so that the numbers can be seen in the dark.

While conducting experiments in his darkened laboratory, he noticed that a fluorescent screen located six feet across his laboratory was glowing. Because Roentgen knew that the cathode rays could travel only short distances in air outside the cathode tube, he realized that he was observing a new, unknown ray, which he called an x ray because the symbol "x" is used for the unknown in mathematics (Fig. 6, V-1).

Roentgen did a series of experiments and discovered many of the properties of x rays. A variety of objects were positioned in the x-ray beam, and images were made on a fluorescent screen. When metal objects such as lead or brass were placed in front of the screen, a shadow of the object appeared on the screen. The metal stopped the x rays, preventing them from reaching the screen, and their shadow was seen. When paper or wood objects were placed in front of the screen, the glow on the screen was

changed only slightly because the x rays were able to pass through these materials quite easily.

While he was positioning one of the objects in the x-ray beam, Roentgen was amazed to see a shadow of the bones of his hand. The x rays were able to penetrate the soft tissues easily, but more x rays were stopped by the harder bone tissue, producing an image of his fingers. In order to find any defects, Roentgen continued to make radiographs, including one of his wife's hand and another of the metal barrel of his shotgun.

The news of the discovery of the x ray spread rapidly throughout the world. The first dental radiograph was taken by Dr. Otto Walkoff in Germany in 1895. He used a small glass plate and an x-ray exposure of 25 minutes. Within ten years x rays were being used for diagnosis of medical and dental conditions, radiation therapy, and scientific studies.

Since the days of the early investigators, x-ray equipment has been improved by many technical advances. The introduction of alternating current allowed the use of higher electrical voltages. The use of a metal target for the cathode rays inside the cathode tube improved the efficiency of the production of x rays and prevented electrical shock to the patient or dental staff. Properly grounded x-ray machines were developed around 1920. By 1986, exposure times had been reduced 15,000 times compared to those used by the early investigators.

RADIATION PHYSICS

Nature of Electromagnetic Radiation

Electromagnetic radiations are various types of energies that are made up of oscillating magnetic and electric fields that travel through space. Radio and television waves, visible light, cosmic rays, and x rays are examples of electromagnetic radiations. Although visible light can be seen by the human eye, other electromagnetic radiations are detected using film (x rays) or radio or television receivers. Electromagnetic radiations have the following properties:

1. *They consist of energy only.* Unlike situations in which work is done by moving matter through space over a distance, such as a bowling ball moving with force to knock over bowling pins, no movement of mass is involved with electromagnetic radiations. Pure energy is transferred through space and is detected electronically or on film.

2. Electromagnetic radiations *travel in straight lines at the speed of light* (186,000 miles per second).

3. Electromagnetic radiations *move through space in the form of transverse waves.* Two types of physical waves are described: longitudinal and transverse. *Longitudinal* waves can be visualized by imagining waves coming into the beach. The wave motion occurs in the same direction in which the water is moving. With *transverse* waves the direction of the wave motion is at right angles to the direction of movement of the energy. This can be visualized by looking at the wave drawn in Figure 7, V-1 and imagining that this represents the wave form of electromagnetic energy. In the case of electromagnetic energy (light or x rays), the energy would be traveling from the page towards the reader and the waves would be moving across the printed page.

The wavelength (λ) is the distance between the peaks of adjacent waves. The wavelength is the characteristic that separates electromagnetic radiations from each other. Examples of radiations with short wavelengths are x rays and cosmic rays. Electromagnetic radiations with longer wavelengths are visible light, radio waves, and television transmissions (Fig. 8, V-1).

Knowledge about electromagnetic radiation is important to the dental radiographer when setting

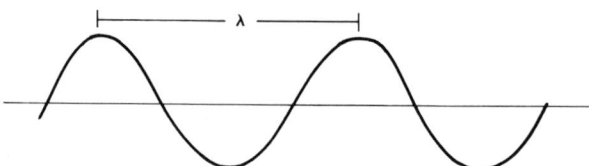

Fig. 7, V-1 Wave motion of electromagnetic radiations. The wavelength λ is measured between peaks of successive waves. Transverse waves (x rays) would be moving from the page toward the reader. Longitudinal waves (sound) would be moving from reader's left to right.

the controls on the x-ray machine to make radiographs. The wavelength of the x-ray beam used to make patient films can be changed by adjusting the kilovolt potential (kVp) setting. When the kVp is higher (70 to 80 kVp), the wavelength of the x rays is decreased and the x rays pass through the patient to the film more easily. Therefore, as higher kVp settings are used, a reduced amount of radiation is needed and shorter exposure times are indicated.

Nature of X rays

X rays are a form of electromagnetic radiation useful in diagnostic radiology because of their ability to penetrate the teeth and jaws. The relatively short wavelength permits the x rays to penetrate materials such as air and soft tissues easily, while more dense objects such as bone, enamel, and dentin absorb the greater portion of the x-ray beam. X rays chemically alter the silver bromide crystals in the film emulsion in such a way that after film processing, an image of the patient is formed on the film.

X rays also affect a fluorescent screen by causing the screen to give off light. The fluorescent material in the intensifying screen has the property of changing x-ray energy to light energy. Not only is this the property that led Dr. Roentgen to the discovery of x rays, but its application in the construction of intensifying screens permits the use of much less radiation during patient examinations. Intensifying screens are installed in cassettes that hold the film during the exposure of extraoral radiographs such as panoramic or cephalometric films. The purpose of the intensifying screens is to change the x-ray energy that passes through the patient into light energy. The film inside the cassette is exposed mostly by the light formed rather than by direct exposure to x rays. This will be discussed in more detail in Section 4.

X rays may also cause injury to biologic tissues. When x rays pass through living tissues, ionization of certain chemicals in the tissues occurs. Some of

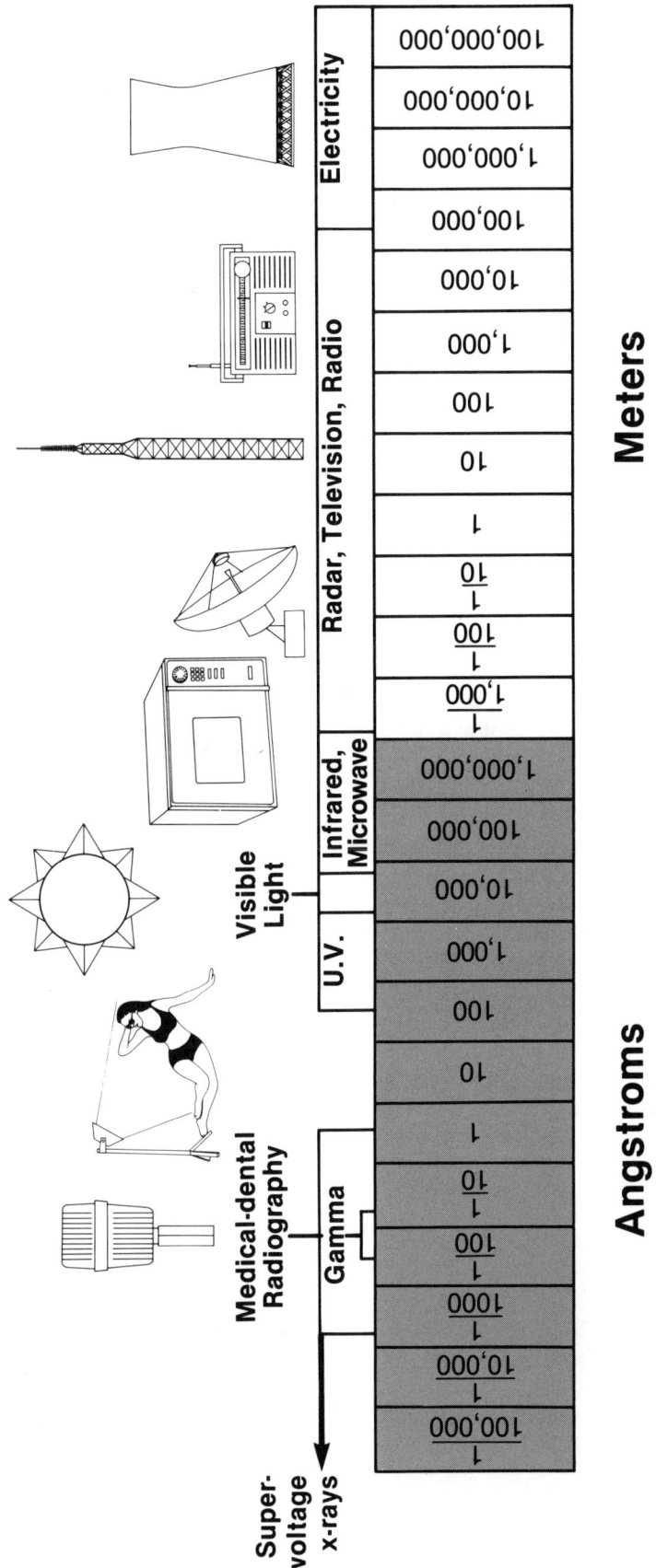

Fig. 8, V-1 Electromagnetic scale.

11

these injuries will heal completely but some permanent damage can take place. This will be discussed in more detail in Section 2.

Production of X rays

In the Crookes tube used by Roentgen, x rays were produced when the rapidly moving electrons hit the gas molecules in the tube or the glass case itself. The impact of the electrons hitting these structures resulted in the production of x rays. In a modern x-ray tube, x rays are produced more efficiently by directing a stream of high-speed electrons against a tungsten target inside the glass tube (Fig. 9, V-1). Following is a list of the parts of the x-ray tube (Fig. 10, V-1):

1. *Metal case*: outer case that contains the x-ray tube and oil-bath chamber. The inside surface of the metal case is covered with a layer of lead that limits the amount of leakage of radiation through the metal case.

2. *Cathode*: negatively charged terminal of the x-ray tube which contains the coiled wire filament from which the electron stream is emitted.

3. *Anode*: positively charged terminal of the x-ray tube consisting of the tungsten target attached to the copper stem.

4. *Target*: tungsten inset into the face of the anode. The electrons are directed from the cathode to hit the face of the tungsten target and x rays are given off from the target. The electrons hit the target on a small impact area called the focal spot.

5. *Heat radiator*: metal bulb that is attached to the copper stem of the anode. Intense heat is given off when the electrons strike the target. Because this heat could cause melting of the target, the heat radiator is installed to conduct the heat away from the target through the copper stem. The radiator itself is cooled by the surrounding oil bath.

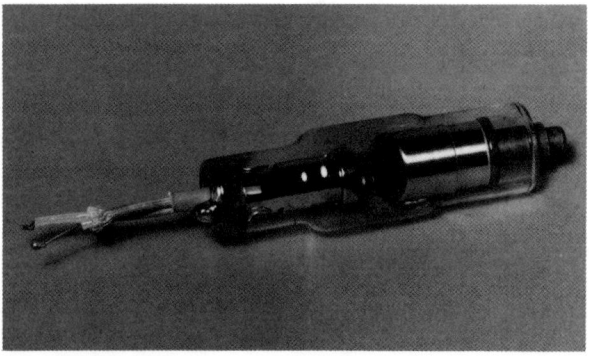

Fig. 9, V-1 Dental x-ray tube. Actual size is approximately 6 in. in length.

6. *Focusing cup*: an inset area that contains the filament in the face of the anode. This device directs the stream of electrons toward the focal spot on the target.

7. *Glass case*: the glass envelope that contains the anode and cathode. Air has been removed from the space inside the glass case, thus creating a vacuum. The vacuum permits the electrons to flow rapidly from the cathode to the anode.

8. *Aperture window*: opening in the glass case through which x rays travel toward the patient.

9. *Collimator (lead diaphragm)*: lead disc with an opening in the center. The collimator limits the size of the x-ray beam that is permitted to pass toward the patient.

10. *Metal filter*: solid disc of metal, usually aluminum, that is placed in the path of the entire x-ray beam. The x-ray beam filter removes the soft x rays (those with low penetrating power) from the x-ray beam.

11. *Kilovolt potential circuit (kVp)*: electrical circuit that connects the anode to the cathode and determines that the cathode is negatively charged and the anode is positively charged. High electrical voltages are required to make x rays and these are formed by a high-voltage transformer that is used in the kVp circuit. The transformers used in a kVp circuit are called step-up transformers because the incoming house voltage of 120 volts is increased to 65,000–90,000 volts needed in the x-ray tube. The kVp settings used in dental x-ray machines vary from 65 to 90. Some dental x-ray machines use preset kVp settings, and other machines permit the operator to change the kVp when needed (variable kVp).

12. *Milliampere circuit (mA)*: electrical circuit that is attached to the cathode and sends electrical current through the filament in the cathode. This current causes heating of the filament, which results in the emission of electrons in the x-ray tube. The milliamperage settings used in dental x-ray machines range from 5 to 15.

X-Ray Generation

X rays are given off when the operator depresses the exposure switch and electricity passes through the milliampere and kilovolt potential circuits. Electrons are emitted from the filament of the cathode in a similar way as occurs in an ordinary light bulb. Current passing through the filament heats the coiled wire to very high temperatures and electrons are given off by a process called *thermionic emission* (Fig. 11A, V-1). The kVp circuit establishes an electrical potential difference between the cathode and an-

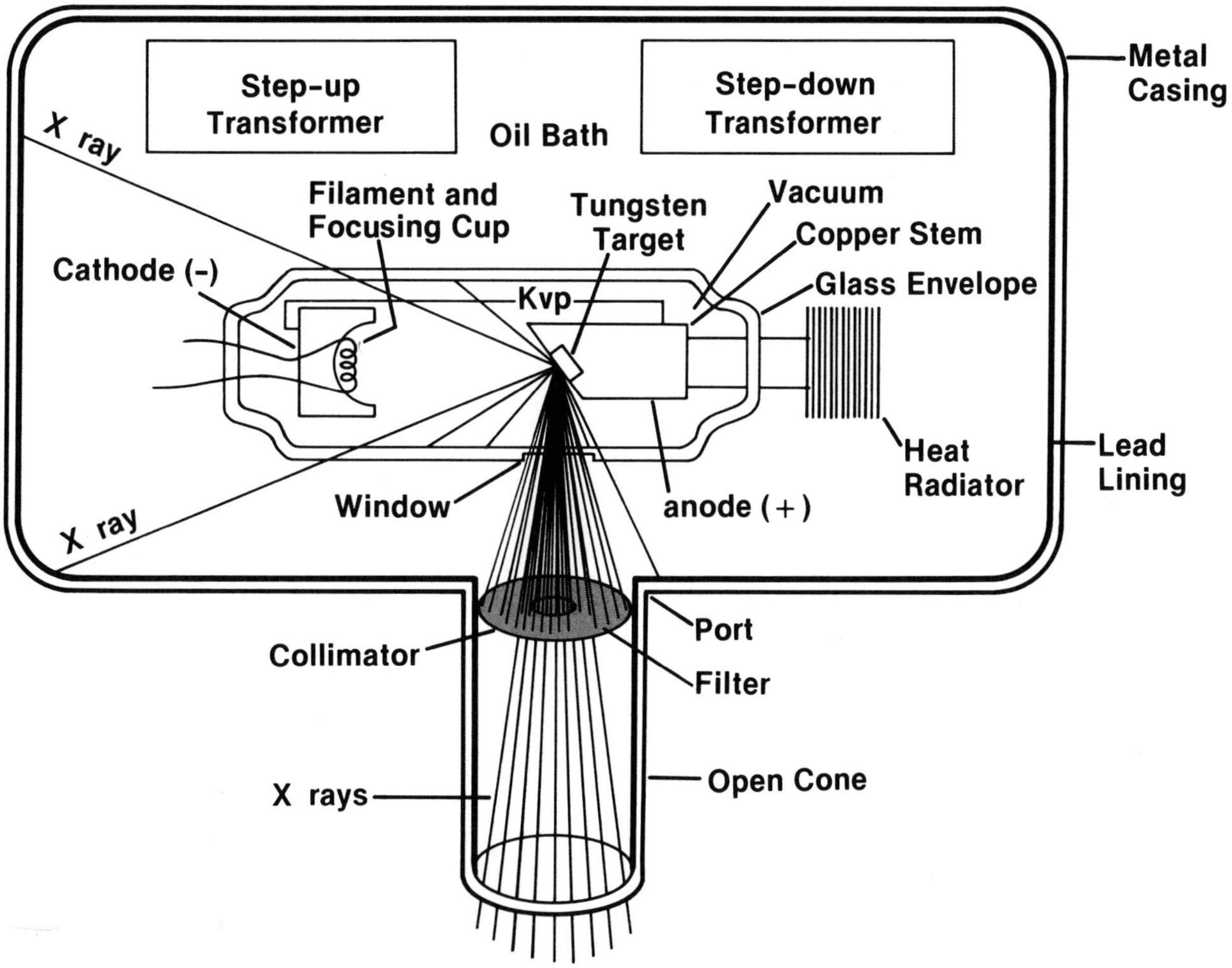

Step-up Transformer   **Oil Bath**   **Step-down Transformer**   **Metal Casing**

X ray

Filament and Focusing Cup   **Tungsten Target**   **Vacuum**   **Copper Stem**   **Glass Envelope**

Cathode (-)   Kvp

X ray

Window   **anode (+)**   **Heat Radiator**   **Lead Lining**

Collimator   **Port**   **Filter**

X rays   **Open Cone**

Fig. 10, V-1 X-ray tubehead. When kVp setting is increased, the electrons are attracted more strongly to the target, resulting in x rays with more penetrating power.

An increased setting in the mA circuit causes the generation of more x rays due to the release of more electrons.

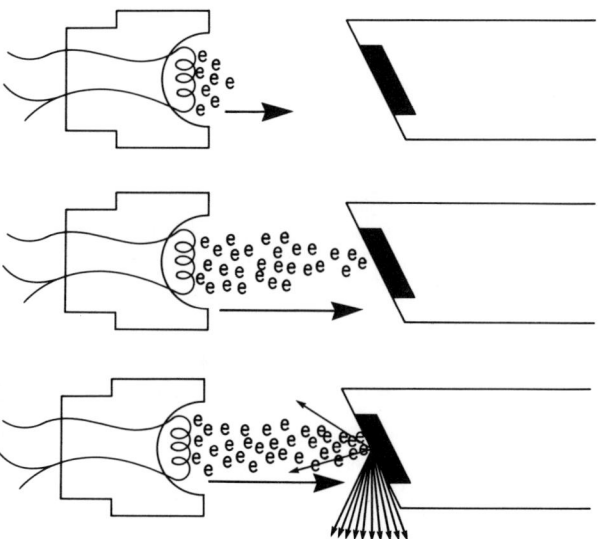

Fig. 11, V-1 A. An x-ray tube showing formation of an electron cloud at the cathode as filament circuit is activated.

B. An x-ray tube showing electrons traveling across the tube from the cathode to anode target as high-voltage circuit is activated by the operator.

C. An x-ray tube showing production of x rays as high-speed electrons collide with the target.

ode of the tube, with the cathode negatively charged and the anode positively charged. Because the electrons are negatively charged particles they are attracted to the positively charged anode terminal at a rapid rate of speed. The direction in which the electrons travel toward the target is controlled by the focusing cup on the face of the cathode. The focusing cup condenses the electrons into a stream that is narrowed to hit the target in an area of about one square millimeter (Fig. 11B, V-1). X rays are produced as a result of the forceful collision of the electrons on the tungsten target, and the x rays are given off in all directions from the target (Fig. 11C, V-1). The useful portion of the beam escapes from within the tube through the aperture and travels to the patient through the cone. The remaining portion of x rays is stopped by the lead lining of the metal case. In addition to x rays being given off, considerable heat is produced in the target. The tubehead is designed to conduct this heat away from the tungsten target to prevent its melting. This is done by inserting the target in a heavy copper cylinder called the stem. Copper is used because it is an excellent conductor of heat, and the heat in the target is transferred from the tungsten to the copper. In addition, a radiator bulb is placed on the end of the stem, which conducts the heat into the oil-bath chamber, thereby protecting the copper stem from overheating.

Two types of x radiation are formed:

1. *Bremsstrahlen radiation*: The fast-moving electrons are stopped rapidly in the central areas of the tungsten atoms in the target. This slowing action of the electrons has been called *bremsstrahlen* (the German word for "rapid braking"). As a result of the interaction of the electrons and tungsten, energy is given off in the form of x rays and heat. The resulting x-ray beam consists of x rays with a broad range of energies, ranging from x rays with poor penetrating ability to those with high penetrating ability. This type of x-ray beam is termed a *polychromatic* beam.

2. *Characteristic radiation*: This is the second type of x ray that is produced at the target. Characteristic radiation consists of specific x-ray energies that are produced when the rapidly moving electrons in the x-ray tube penetrate the tungsten atom and directly strike the electrons located in the innermost electron shell of the tungsten atoms. Instead of the wide range of x rays produced during the *bremsstrahlen* reaction, x rays of specific energies are produced, which in the case of tungsten is 68 or 58 kVp. This type of x-ray beam is termed a *monochromatic* beam.

The useful x-ray beam is composed of both *bremsstrahlen* and characteristic radiations; however, most of the beam is made up of general, broad-spectrum radiation formed by the *bremsstrahlen* mechanism.

OPERATION OF THE DENTAL X-RAY MACHINE

Components of the X-Ray Machine

CONSOLE. The console contains the circuit boards and controls that enable the operator to set the correct exposure techniques for patient examinations (timer, mA, and kVp). An "on-off" switch must be positioned in the "on" position to operate the equipment. The timer dial is marked with time intervals, and the correct timer setting is set by turning the dial to the correct position. The mA control (buttons or a dial) permits the operator to set the correct mA. The kVp setting is made by turning the kVp knob until the correct setting is shown on the kVp meter (Fig. 12A, V-1). Some manufacturers fix the mA and the kVp on the x-ray machine at the factory, and if that type of equipment is used, it is not necessary to make these settings manually.

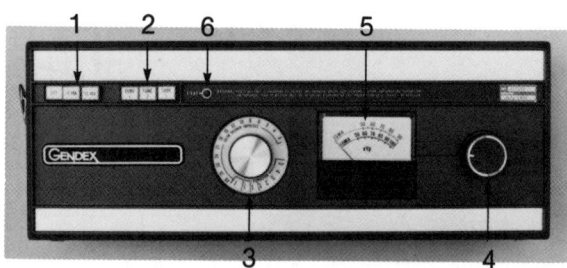

Fig. 12, V-1 A. X-ray machine console. (1) mA setting and on-off switch, (2) tubehead selector switches, (3) time setting, (4) kVp selector, (5) kVp meter, and (6) x-ray exposure light. *(Courtesy of Gendex Corp., Milwaukee, WI)*

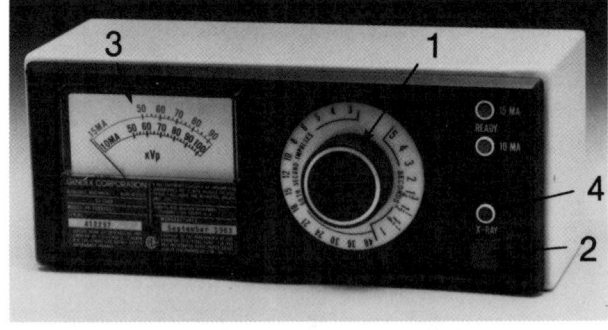

B. Remote station controls timer settings and exposure for individual x-ray room. (1) timer, (2) exposure switch, (3) kVp meter, and (4) x-ray exposure light. *(Courtesy of Gendex Corp., Milwaukee, WI)*

Some consoles are capable of operating more than one x-ray tubehead. These are made available by manufacturers to provide an economic way to equip large dental offices with x-ray machines in a number of dental operatories. When multiple tubeheads are controlled by the console, a device called a "remote station" is installed outside the doorway of the operatory. Each remote station consists of an exposure switch, a timer dial, and a kVp meter. Use of the remote station allows the operator to expose films for each operatory while being close enough to observe the patient during the exposure (Fig. 12B, V-1).

The exposure switch activates the machine to produce x rays. The operator must depress the button firmly and hold it down until the complete preset exposure is completed. An exposure light on the console will be illuminated during x-ray exposure. The machine will not be activated a second time until the switch is released entirely and depressed a second time.

Dental x-ray equipment varies considerably in design and installation. Therefore, the dental x-ray operator must become familiar with the specific installation and operating procedures in the dental office; otherwise inadvertent exposure of patients and personnel may occur.

TUBEHEAD AND ARM ASSEMBLY. The tubehead and arm assembly are firmly attached to the wall of the dental operatory (Fig. 13, V-1). The flexible extension arm allows the tubehead to be positioned in the varied positions required for dental radiography. The tubehead contains the x-ray tube with surrounding oil bath and metal case. An extension cone is placed on the tubehead to direct the position of the x-ray beam and set the correct distance from the tubehead to the patient.

X-Ray Machine Settings

An important factor in making high-quality radiographs is the production of films with good image density (blackness) and contrast (distinct white and black shades). The correct setting of the controls on the x-ray console is important for enhancing both contrast and density. To establish the machine settings correctly, the following should be taken into consideration:

KVP: The kVp setting affects the image contrast and density. Image contrast is the difference between the white and black shadows on the film. An image that has stark white and dark black shadows is described as a high-contrast image. A low-contrast image is seen with many grey tones with the whites not as

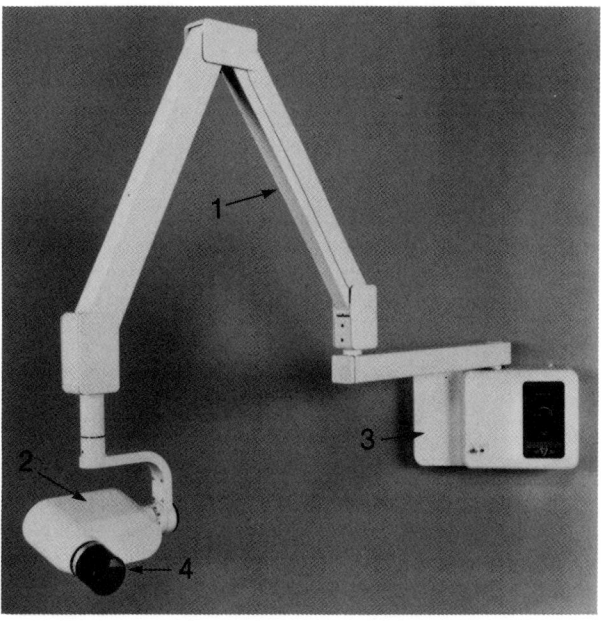

Fig. 13, V-1 Flexible arm and tubehead. (1) flexible arm, (2) tubehead, (3) control box, and (4) cone. *(Courtesy of Gendex Corp., Milwaukee, WI)*

white or the blacks as black as those in high contrast-images (Fig. 14, V-1). High kVp (90 kVp) settings result in low-contrast images and low kVp (70 kVp) settings result in high-contrast images. When higher kVp techniques are used, lower mAs settings are required because the x-ray beam is more penetrating than when a lower kVp is used.

MA AND TIME SETTINGS. The quantity of radiation output of the x-ray machine is determined by the mA and time settings and is calculated by multiplying the mA × time(seconds) = mAs (milliampere seconds). From this equation it is evident that the mA and timer settings are inversely proportional (as mA increases, the timer setting decreases). A common procedure used in dental offices is to set the mA at the highest figure available on that machine and then establish the correct timer setting. This technique results in the use of shorter time settings, which is helpful in avoiding patient motion artifacts on the radiographs. The mA and timer settings are established taking into account the speed of the film being used, the length of the cone installed on the tubehead, and the size and condition of the patient.

1. *Film speed.* Intraoral dental film is available in two film speeds: Ultraspeed and Ektaspeed (Eastman Kodak Co.). If the faster film is used (Ektaspeed), the mAs settings should be reduced. See Figure 15A, B, V-1. Note that the time settings for the

70 kVp
10 MA
36 Impulses

90 kVp
10 MA
20 Impulses

Fig. 14, V-1 Example of contrast scales. Low kVp (70)=high contrast. High kVp (90)=low contrast.

Ektaspeed chart are reduced to approximately 50 percent of those used with the slower Ultraspeed film.

2. *Cone length.* The extension cone on the x-ray tubehead establishes the distance from the tubehead to the patient. This distance must be taken into account when establishing the correct mA and timer settings. The relationship between the distance and the intensity of the x-ray beam follows the *inverse square law.* The law states: *The intensity of the beam of x rays varies inversely as the square of the distance from the x-ray source to the film* (Fig. 16, V-1). mAs settings are established for each cone length. Any change in cone length dictates an adjustment to the mAs setting: use of a longer cone will require an increase in mAs, and the use of a shorter cone, less mAs. See Figure 15, V-1. Note that for each set of time figures, a 16-in. cone requires *four* times greater exposure time than an 8-in. cone.

3. *Patient size.* Exposure guidelines usually indicate that for children exposure be reduced by one-third, for edentulous patients it be reduced by one-quarter, and for large adults the mAs be increased by 10 percent.

BIBLIOGRAPHY

Curry, T. S., III; Dowdey, J. E.; and Murry, R. C., Jr. *Christensen's Physics of Diagnostic Radiology.* 4th ed. Philadelphia: Lea & Febiger, 1990.

De Lyre, W. R., and Johnson, O. N. *Essentials of Dental Radiography for Dental Assistants and Hygienists.* 4th ed. Norwalk, Conn.: Appleton & Lange, 1990.

Eastman Kodak Company. *X-Rays in Dentistry.* Rochester, N.Y.: Radiology Markets Division, 1985.

Frommer, H. H. *Radiology for Dental Auxiliaries.* 4th ed. St. Louis: C. V. Mosby Co., 1987.

Langland, O. E.; Langlais, R. P.; Sippy, F. H.; and Williamson, G. *Radiology for Dental Hygienists and Dental Assistants.* Springfield, Ill.: Charles C. Thomas, 1988.

Langland, O. E.; Sippy, F.; and Langlais, R. P. *Textbook of Dental Radiology.* 2d ed. Springfield, Ill.: Charles C. Thomas, 1984.

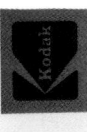

EXPOSURE GUIDELINES
for KODAK Ultra-Speed Dental X-ray Film

Exposure Factors		65 kV 10 mA		70 kV 10 mA		80 kV 10 mA		90 kV 10 mA		FACTORS FOR THIS OFFICE				
Patient		Adult*		Adult*		Adult*		Adult*		kV			mA	
										Adult		Child		
Source-Image Distance		8″	16″	8″	16″	8″	16″	8″	16″	8″	16″	8″	16″	
Region	Vertical Angle	APPROXIMATE EXPOSURE IN IMPULSES												
Maxillary														
Incisor	+40°	15	60	12	48	7	28	5	20					
Cuspid	+45°	15	60	12	48	7	28	5	20					
Bicuspid	+30°	19	76	15	60	9	36	6	24					
Molar	+20°	22	88	18	72	10	40	7	28					
Mandibular														
Incisor	−15°	12	48	9	36	5	20	4	16					
Cuspid	−20°	12	48	9	36	5	20	4	16					
Bicuspid	−10°	13	52	11	44	6	24	5	20					
Molar	− 5°	15	60	12	48	7	28	5	20					
Anterior Bite-Wing														
Type 1 Adult	+ 8°	12	48	9	36	5	20	4	16					
Type 1 Child	+ 8°	*	*	*	*	*	*	*	*					
Posterior Bite-Wing														
Type 2 or 3 Adult	+ 8°	15	60	12	48	7	28	5	20					
Type 0 Child	+ 8°													

*Children: Reduce adult exposure time about one-third.   Edentulous areas: Reduce exposure time about one-quarter.

The above guidelines were developed following recommended time-temperature processing with Kodak chemicals. Method to compute mAs or mAi: mAs is the product of milliamperage times seconds of exposure. mAi is the product of milliamperage times the impulses of energy. If the product is the same in either case, the quantity of radiation produced is essentially the same.

Examples: mA × sec = mAs; mA × imp = mAi
10 × 1/2 = 5 ; 10 × 30 = 300
15 × 1/3 = 5 ; 15 × 20 = 300

IF 15 mA IS USED INSTEAD OF 10 mA—REDUCE EXPOSURE FACTOR BY ONE-THIRD

CONVERSION CHART

Fractions	Decimals	Impulses
1/60		1
1/30		2
1/20	0.05	3
1/15		4
1/12	0.10	5
1/10		6
1/8		8
2/15	0.15	9
3/20		10
1/6	0.20	12
1/5	0.25	15
1/4		15
4/15	0.30	18
3/10		20
1/3	0.35	21
7/20	0.40	24
3/8		
2/5	0.45	27
5/12		
9/20	0.50	30
7/15		
1/2	0.55	33
8/15		
11/20	0.60	36
7/12		
3/5	0.65	39
5/8		40
13/20	0.70	42
2/3		
7/10	0.75	45
11/15	0.80	48
3/4	0.85	51
4/5		
17/20		
13/15		
7/8		
9/10	0.90	54
11/12		
14/15		
19/20	0.95	57
1	1.00	60
1-1/4	1.25	75
1-1/2	1.50	90

EASTMAN KODAK COMPANY
Health Sciences Markets Division • Rochester, N.Y. 14650

KODAK is a trademark.

MTS-7—4-82
T.M. REG. U.S. PAT. OFF
© EASTMAN KODAK COMPANY. 1982

Fig. 15, V-1 A. Exposure guidelines for Ultra-Speed Dental X-ray Film. (*Reprinted courtesy of Eastman Kodak Co., Rochester, NY*)

EXPOSURE GUIDELINES
for KODAK *EKTASPEED* Dental X-ray Film

APPROXIMATE EXPOSURE IN IMPULSES

Exposure Factors		65 kV 10 mA Adult*		70 kV 10 mA Adult*		80 kV 10 mA Adult*		90 kV 10 mA Adult*		FACTORS FOR THIS OFFICE					
Patient										kV	mA	Adult		Child	
Source-Image Distance	Vertical Angle	8″	16″	8″	16″	8″	16″	8″	16″	8″	16″	8″	16″	8″	16″
Maxillary Incisor	+40°	8	30	6	24	4	14	N	10						
Cuspid	+45°	8	30	6	24	4	14	O	10						
Bicuspid	+30°	10	38	8	30	5	18	T	12						
Molar	+20°	11	44	9	36	5	20	R	14						
Mandibular Incisor	−15°	6	24	5	18	3	10	E	8						
Cuspid	−20°	6	24	5	18	3	10	C	8						
Bicuspid	−10°	7	26	6	22	3	12	O	10						
Molar	−5°	8	30	6	24	4	14	M	10						
Anterior Bite-Wing Type 1 Adult	+8°	6	24	5	18	3	10	M E N	8						
Type 1 Child	+8°	*	*	*	*	*	*	.	.						
Posterior Bite-Wing Type 2 or 3 Adult	+8°	8	30	6	24	4	14	D E	10						
Type 0 Child	+8°	*	*	*	*	*	*	D	.						

(The 90 kV 8″ column reads vertically: "NOT RECOMMENDED".)

IF 15 mA IS USED INSTEAD OF 10 mA—REDUCE EXPOSURE FACTOR BY ONE-THIRD

CONVERSION CHART

Fractions	Decimals	Impulses
1/60		1
1/30		2
1/20	0.05	3
1/15		4
1/12		5
1/10	0.10	6
1/8		
2/15		8
3/20	0.15	9
1/6		10
1/5	0.20	12
1/4	0.25	15
4/15		16
3/10	0.30	18
1/3		20
7/20	0.35	21
3/8		
2/5	0.40	24
5/12		
9/20	0.45	27
7/15		28
1/2	0.50	30
8/15		
11/20	0.55	33
7/12		
3/5	0.60	36
13/20	0.65	39
2/3		40
7/10	0.70	42
11/15		
3/4	0.75	45

*Children: Reduce adult exposure time about one-third.   Edentulous areas: Reduce exposure time about one-quarter.

To avoid fractional impulses, some 8″ exposure times have been rounded off to whole numbers. Mathematically, these 8″ times will not comply with the inverse square law in relation to the 16″ exposure times.

The above guidelines were developed following recommended time-temperature processing with Kodak chemicals. Method to compute mAs or mAi: mAs is the product of milliamperage times seconds of exposure. mAi is the product of milliamperage times the impulses of energy. If the product is the same in either case, the quantity of radiation produced is essentially the same.

Examples: mA×sec = mAs; mA×imp = mAi
10×1/2 = 5 ; 10×30 = 300
15×1/3 = 5 ; 15×20 = 300

EASTMAN KODAK COMPANY
Health Sciences Markets Division • Rochester, N.Y. 14650

KODAK and EKTASPEED are trademarks.

MTS-7—4-82
T.M. REG. U.S. PAT. OFF.
©EASTMAN KODAK COMPANY. 1982

B. Exposure guidelines for Ektaspeed Dental X-ray Film. (*Reprinted courtesy of Eastman Kodak Co., Rochester, NY*)

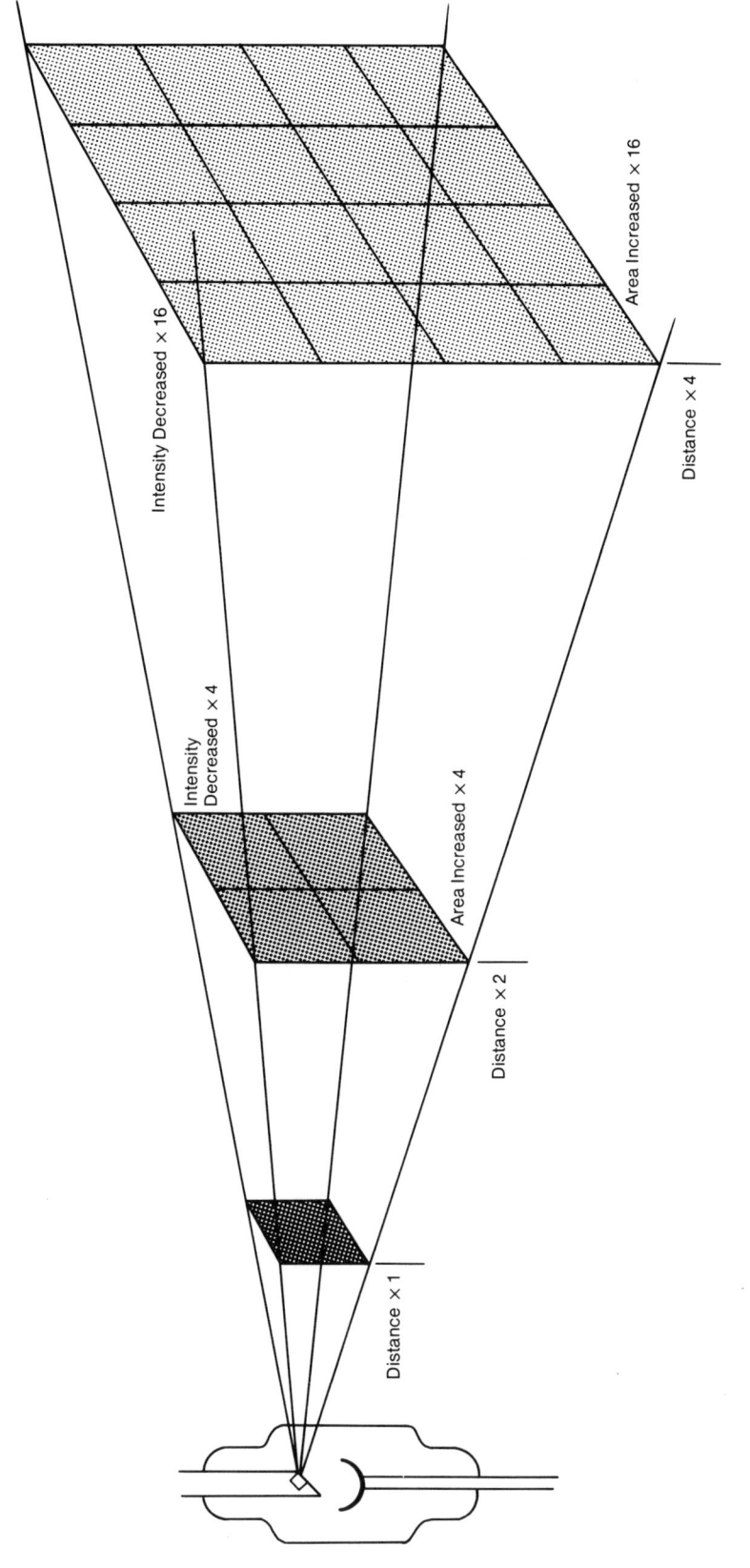

Fig. 16, V-1 Inverse square law. The intensity of the x-ray beam decreases with the square of the distance. The size of the beam increases by the square of the distance.

19

Section 1

Examination

I. In answering the following questions, write the answer in the space below the question.

The radiographic density of silver restorations is (1).

1. _____

Examples of substances in the oral cavity that are radiolucent are (2) and (3).

2. _____

3. _____

Why is the pulp tissue radiolucent on the film?

4. _____

Caries is radiolucent on a radiograph because (5).

5. _____

Destruction of the alveolar bone around the apex of a tooth is characteristic of (6) disease.

6. _____

The dental auxiliary's ability to (7) and (8) is an asset that is valuable to the dentist.

7. _____

8. _____

Three characteristics of cathode rays are (9), (10), and (11).

9. _____

10. _____

11. _____

What made Roentgen realize that he was observing a new ray when the fluorescent screen glowed in his laboratory?

12. _____

Three characteristics of electromagnetic radiations are (13), (14), and (15).

13. _____

14. _____

15. _____

Three characteristics of x rays are (16), (17), and (18).

16. _____

17. _____

18. _____

II. Answer the following questions on a separate sheet of paper.

1. Draw a diagram of the dental x-ray tubehead and label the following: cathode, anode, target, heat radiator, focusing cup, glass case, aperture window, collimator, aluminum filter, kVp circuit, and mA circuit.

2. List the steps involved in x-ray generation in a modern dental x-ray tube.

3. What is the function of the console of the x-ray machine?

4. What is the purpose of the aluminum filter?

5. What is the purpose of the collimator?

6. The dentist decides to use 90 kVp and 10 mA to expose bitewing films. Using ultraspeed film and a 16-in. cone, what machine settings should be used to take films on adults? Use Fig. 15, V-1 to answer this question.

7. The dentist decides to use 70 kVp and 10 mA to expose bitewing films. Using Ektaspeed film and an 8-in. cone, what machine settings should be used to take films on adults? Use Fig. 15, V-1 to answer this question.

8. If an 8-in. cone is replaced by a 16-in. cone and other factors are kept the same, the time setting should be changed by what factor?

9. When children are being radiographed, by how much should the exposure be adjusted?

10. When edentulous patients are being radiographed, by how much should the exposure be adjusted?

Radiation Biology and Protection

The dental radiographer is called upon to expose patients with radiation for diagnostic purposes. An understanding of the potential hazards associated with radiation exposure is essential to complete the radiographic examination with minimum risk to the patient and the operator. This section describes the radiation effects associated with low doses of x rays and provides technical procedures used to limit exposure to the safest practical levels.

OBJECTIVES

1. To describe the mechanism of tissue damage resulting from x radiation.
2. To compare genetic and somatic effects of radiation.
3. To compare direct and indirect effects of radiation.
4. To list and explain four effects of radiation on cells.
5. To explain the differences in radiation sensitivity demonstrated by different cells.
6. To describe the chronic effects of low-level radiation on tissues and organs.
7. To list two sites in the head and neck that are sensitive to radiation and discuss methods of reducing their exposure during dental radiography.
8. To explain how radiation effects are accumulated.
9. To define radiation protection terms.
10. To list and describe six procedures used to protect the patient from unnecessary radiation exposure.
11. To list and describe six procedures used to protect the x-ray machine operator from unnecessary x-ray exposure.

RADIATION BIOLOGY

Mechanism of Tissue Damage

Ionization of the molecules of living tissues is the basic mechanism of tissue damage resulting from exposure to x rays. Ionization occurs when the atoms of a molecule are separated into charged atomic particles. For example, common table salt, sodium chloride ($NaCl$), is ionized when it is dissolved in water as the sodium and chloride atoms separate into ($Na+$) and chloride ($Cl-$) ions ($NaCl \rightarrow Na+ + Cl-$). When x rays are absorbed by the tissues, the molecules of the tissues are ionized and damage may result.

Genetic and Somatic Effects

Radiation exposure to the reproductive organs of adults of child-bearing age may result in the absorption of x rays by the reproductive cells. This can result in alterations in the genetic code of these cells and possibly lead to radiation-induced mutations (sudden changes in an inherited characteristic) in the offspring. This type of effect in subsequent generations is called the *genetic effect. Somatic effects* are those that are expressed in the exposed person rather than in the offspring, such as radiation burns on the skin of the exposed person.

Direct and Indirect Effects of Radiation

There are two types of biological effects caused by x rays: direct and indirect. *Direct effects* are caused by direct interaction between the x rays and a specific target in the cell such as the nucleus or cell membrane. The direct effect is usually applied to the explanation of radiation effects on dry plant systems such as spores and seeds.

The *indirect effect* is the most usual effect that occurs in animals, including people, and it describes the reaction between x rays and the water molecules that comprise a large percentage of animal tissues. The water molecules (H_2O) are ionized to hydrogen (H_2) and oxygen (O_2) atoms, which recombine into chemical groupings of these two atoms called *radicals*; for example, hydrogen peroxide (H_2O_2) or hydroxyl (OH_2). These radicals cause the actual chemical damage to the tissues and cells. This effect is termed indirect because the x rays ionize the water and the recombined hydrogen and oxygen ions cause the actual damage. These radicals form immediately upon x-ray exposure and are present in the tissues and cells for only a fraction of a second since they quickly reform into water. The damage that results from x-ray exposure is initiated during that brief fraction of time that the radicals are active in the tissues.

Radiation Effects on Cells

A cell is the small biological unit of the body and consists of the central nucleus, surrounding cytoplasm, and an outer cell wall. The body is composed of many types of cells, muscle, nerve, and blood, which perform the various required biological functions. Radiation effects upon cells can be any of the following:

1. *Cell death*. If sufficiently high doses of x rays are absorbed by a cell, immediate or delayed death of the cell may occur.

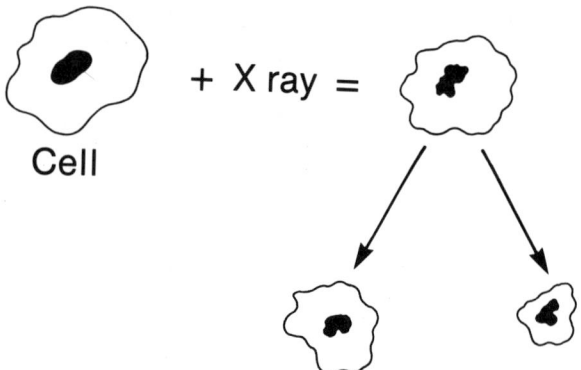

Fig. 1, V-2 Aberration during cell division. Daughter cells of radiated cell are different in size of cell and nucleus.

2. *Swelling of the cell*. Radiation can impair the normal interchange of fluid through the cell wall and result in an increase in the size of the cell.

3. *Change in cell function*. Radiation can result in alterations in the specific function of the individual cell, such as the production of a protein or enzyme of changed chemical composition. These changes alter the physiologic actions of these cell products.

4. *Aberration in cell division*. Radiation can result in improper events during the division of a cell such that the daughter cells are different in some way from the parent cell. For example, one daughter cell may be larger or smaller than its paired cell, or other inherited traits may be unevenly proportioned between the two offspring cells (Fig. 1, V-2).

Sensitivity of Cells to Radiation

All cells of the body are not equally susceptible to radiation. Those cells that are more sensitive to x rays, that is, more likely to be affected by radiation, are immature, rapidly dividing, and do not perform specialized functions. Cells are more susceptible to radiation during cell division, which explains why rapidly dividing immature cells are more sensitive.

Examples of more sensitive cells are:

1. Basal cells of the skin that divide rapidly and replenish the outer skin layers that are continually sloughed and replaced. This is the basis for the development of skin cancer due to prolonged exposure to x ray or sunlight.

2. Bone marrow cells, which are the precursors of all circulating red and white blood cells. The high turnover of bone marrow cells continues throughout life due to the continuing need for the renewal of these blood cells. This is the basis of the development of leukemia in some individuals who have been exposed to high levels of radiation such as those exposed from atomic weapons or laboratory accidents.

3. All cells in the developing embryo. This is the reason that the embryo is very sensitive to x ray and other irritants.

Cells that tend to be least sensitive to radiation are well-differentiated, mature, functioning cells that rarely undergo cell division, such as nerve, muscle, brain, and circulating red and white blood cells.

Radiation Effects on Tissues and Organs

The cells of the body are organized into larger functioning units—tissues and organs—and their collective sensitivity to radiation is determined by the susceptibility of the cells contained in that tissue or organ. The effect of low doses of x rays on adult tissues and organs is considered to be similar to premature aging. Adult tissues and organs are composed mostly of well-differentiated cells that are performing the function required of that organ; for example, kidney cells filter wastes from the blood, muscle cells contract, and nerve cells transmit nervous impulses. The most sensitive component, or weakest link, of the organ or tissue is the endothelial cells that line the capillary walls. Radiation exposure of the capillary walls may result in swelling of the endothelial cells in the capillary walls, thus preventing the proper flow of blood, and this may affect the integrity of the capillary network. With repeated exposures the functional efficiency of the capillary beds throughout the organ is impaired, resulting not only in a *decrease in performance of tissue functions* but also in a *decrease in defense against infections* and a *decrease in the ability to repair following injury.*

Repair and Accumulation of Radiation Effects

Fortunately, most of the damage caused by low levels of radiation is repaired within the cells, tissues, and organs of the body. Damaging effects of a single exposure to x rays may repair completely. Chronic and repeated exposure to radiation, however, may lead to a minor percentage of unrepaired effects that accumulate in the exposed tissues. The accumulation of radiation effects tends to accelerate the normal aging process in the tissues and organs. Repeated exposures increase the likelihood of an increased number of effects, and higher doses of radiation result in a more rapid expression of the effects.

High doses of radiation can cause immediate effects on the tissues, such as skin reddening or burn. Lower doses of radiation do not result in immediate effects and, in general, as the dose is reduced, the longer the period before an effect occurs. The period of time that elapses between the moment of exposure to the development of the biological effect is called the *latent period*. Early aging, the development of thyroid cancer, and cataract formation in the lens of the eye are examples of effects that develop after a latent period of many years. These effects are caused by high doses of x rays and it is very unlikely that exposure from dental x-ray machines can cause these effects.

Radiation-Sensitive Tissues in the Dental Region

The thyroid gland and the lens of the eye are tissues that are especially sensitive to radiation. Because of their location adjacent to dental areas, they may be exposed to the primary beam of x rays during the exposure of dental radiographs. Thyroid carcinoma has been caused by x rays, although from x-ray doses much higher than those used in dental radiography. Cataracts can be caused by radiation of the eye, but again, the x-ray dose required to cause this effect is much higher than that used in dentistry.

Even though x-ray doses used in dental radiographic procedures are unlikely to cause one of these serious effects, the additive nature of radiation effects from all sources of radiation dictates that all diagnostic radiographic procedures be accomplished using the least amount of radiation possible. The ALARA (as low as reasonably achievable) concept of radiation protection is used by all persons whose occupations require the use of radiation, such as the dentist and dental auxiliary. Dental personnel should take all reasonable measures to restrict the exposure of patients and occupational workers to the least amount of radiation. The use of the paralleling intraoral periapical technique is an example of a method available for dental radiography that enables the operator to obtain films while reducing exposure to the eye and thyroid gland. The vertical angulation used in this technique is less steep than that employed in the bisecting-the-angle technique, and thereby reduces the amount of radiation that strikes the eye and thyroid gland. The use of a beam collimated intraoral technique results in additional exposure reduction to the head and neck (see pp. 97-107). A thyroid shield is also available to protect the thyroid gland from direct exposure during the exposure of intraoral and cephalometric films. The thyroid shield contains lead material that absorbs the radiation and prevents exposure of the thyroid gland (Fig. 2, V-2).

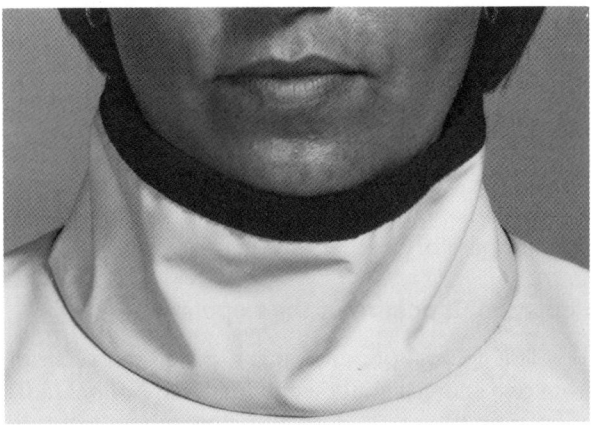

Fig. 2, V-2 Lead apron incorporating a thyroid shield extension to protect the thyroid gland from x-ray exposure.

RADIATION PROTECTION

Terminology

1. Units of measure:

a. *Roentgen (R)* is that amount of x radiation that will ionize 1 cubic centimeter (cc) of air. The roentgen is a physicist's term for measuring the quantities of x rays at the surface of objects.

b. *Roentgen Absorbed Dose (RAD)* is the amount of x radiation that is absorbed in a substance. The biologist uses the RAD to measure the quantities of radiation absorbed in volumes of tissue.

c. *Roentgen Equivalent Man (REM)* is the dose of any ionizing that will produce the same biological effect in man as that produced from the absorption of 1R of x or gamma radiation.

Note that several new terms are replacing the items described above.

New Terms	Old Terms
Coulomb per kilogram	Roentgen
1 c/kg	= 3.88 × 10 R
Gray	Radiation absorbed dose
1 Gy	= 100 RADS
Sievert	Roentgen Equivalent Man
1 Sv	= 100 REM

2. *Primary Radiation*: The x-ray beam that is given off directly by the target of the x-ray machine. Primary radiation consists of high-energy x rays with the intended capability of penetrating substances and ionizing the molecules of tissues. Only the patient being radiographed should be placed in the path of the primary radiation, and the x-ray machine operator should always be stationed in a location that cannot be reached by the primary beam.

3. *Useful Beam*: The radiation that is permitted to emerge from the x-ray machine. The size and shape of the useful beam is determined by the collimator. The x-ray beam is shaped in the form of an expanding cone that enlarges as it passes outwardly from the source of x-rays.

4. *Secondary Radiation* (scatter radiation): The x rays that are formed when the primary rays strike the patient and are scattered in all directions in the dental operatory.

Radiation Exposure of the Population

The general population is exposed to radiation from two sources, natural and artificial. *Natural* radiation from the earth, sun, and atmosphere exposes individuals to about 100 milliroentgen (mR) per year. *Artificial* sources of radiation include diagnostic and therapeutic radiation as well as that associated with atomic testing and scientific experimentation. The major portion of artificial radiation exposure of the public is the result of medical and dental diagnostic radiography. X-ray exposure from diagnostic medical and dental radiographs results in doses of radiation that average 100 milliroentgen per person in the population. This level of radiation is approximately equal to radiation that is present in the normal environment from underground and atmospheric sources (natural background radiation). Because any exposure to x rays carries with it a risk of genetic or somatic injury, all reasonable and practical measures should be employed to prevent all but necessary radiation exposure to the population.

It is of particular importance to observe all measures of patient protection procedures when it is necessary to radiograph a pregnant woman. The developing tissues of the embryo are especially sensitive to radiation because of their rapid growth. A lead apron should be placed over the abdomen of pregnant women during dental radiographic exposures to protect the embryo from scatter radiation.

In the dental office both the patient and the machine operator are subject to x-ray exposure during radiographic examinations, and the following procedures are designed to minimize exposure to both the patient and the office personnel.

Patient Protection

1. Correct radiographic technique during the preparation of dental radiographs eliminates the need to retake films. The dental radiographer must adopt an attitude of "doing it right the first time" to prevent the unnecessary radiation exposure that accompanies retaking films.

2. Using proper film processing procedures in the darkroom is very important with respect to limiting the amount of exposure needed to make the films. The "time-temperature" method of film processing should be employed to process routine radiographs, or an automatic processor should be used. See Section 4.

3. Placement of a protective lead apron over the patient's lap during intraoral radiography (Fig. 3A, V-2) and over the patient's back during panoramic radiography prevents scatter radiation from reaching the patient's reproductive areas (Fig. 3B, V-2).

4. The use of film-holding devices for stabilizing the periapical packets, instead of the out-dated procedure of having patients hold the film with their fingers, eliminates the unnecessary exposure of the patient's hands.

5. The use of proper equipment:

a. *Filtration.* Beam filtration is accomplished by

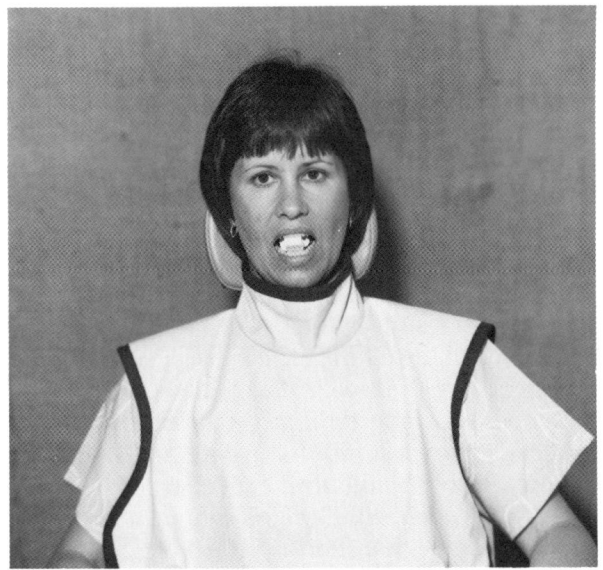

Fig. 3, V-2 A. Lead apron in place for intraoral radiography.

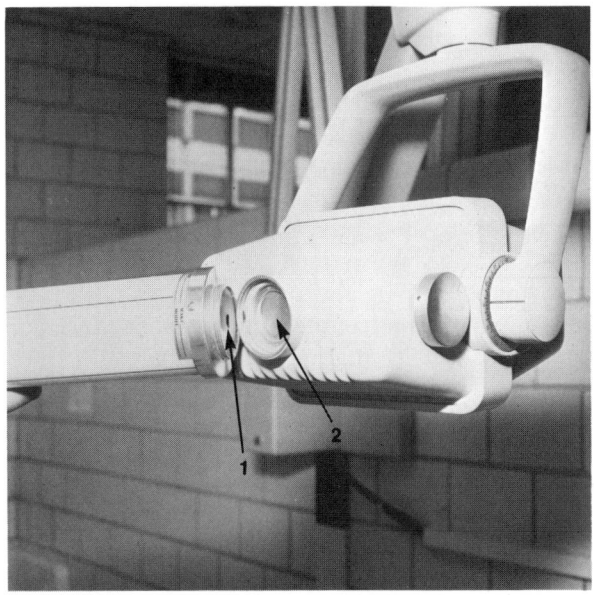

Fig. 4, V-2 A. Tubehead with cone unattached to show: (1) collimator and (2) aluminum filter.

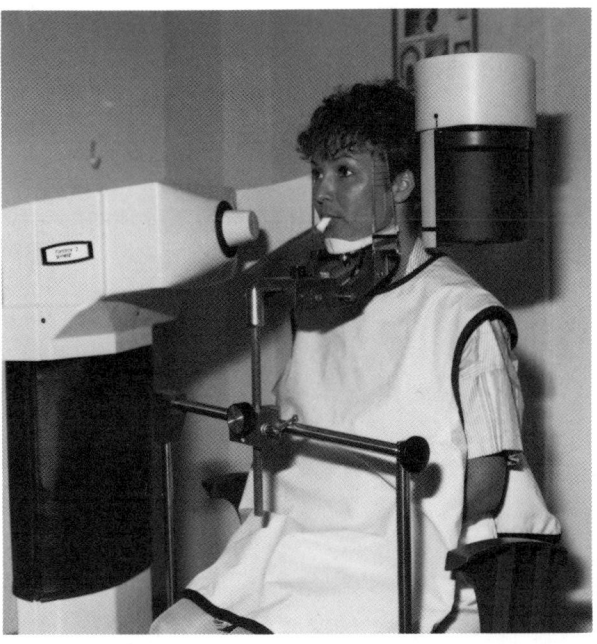

B. Lead apron behind patient during exposure of panoramic films.

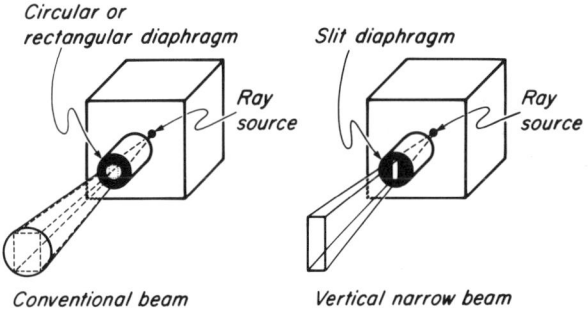

B. Slit collimator used with panoramic x-ray machines.

the installation of a thin aluminum disk in the path of the x-ray beam. The filter is installed at the factory and positioned in the port in the side of the tubehead adjacent to the attachment of the dental x-ray cone (Fig. 4A, V-2). The aluminum filter removes the non-penetrating portion of the x-ray beam, which would be absorbed by the patient's skin and cheek.

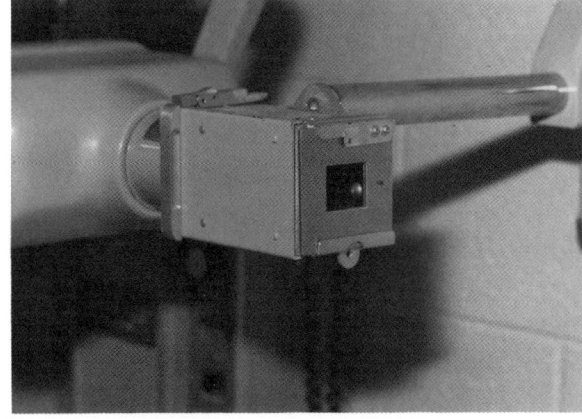

C. Fixator collimator used for cephalometric films to center x-ray beam and reduce size of beam to that of 8-in. × 10-in. cassette.

The filtered beam contains x rays that are more likely to pass through the teeth and alveolar bone forming the image on the film. The thickness of the filter is regulated by state and federal laws. Federal standards indicate that the filter is to be 1.5 mm if an x-ray machine operates at or below 70 kVp, and 2.5 mm if the machine is operated above 70 kVp.

b. *Collimation*. The restriction of the size of the useful x-ray beam is termed beam collimation. This is accomplished by the installation of a lead diaphragm in the path of the x-ray beam. Dental collimators are usually attached in the tubehead end of the cone. The purpose of the collimator is to establish as small a useful beam as is necessary to expose the film. The use of a beam that is larger than the size of the film or film cassette exposes the patient to unnecessary radiation. The collimator used for intraoral radiography is illustrated in Figure 4A, V-2. Additional collimation in intraoral radiography may be provided by using either a rectangular x-ray cone (Rinn Corp.) or the Precision Instrument (Isaac Masel Corp.). See Section 5. Two other types of collimators are used in dentistry: a slit collimator for panoramic x-ray machines (Fig. 4B, V-2) and a special use collimator for cephalometric radiographs for orthodontic and pediatric patients (Fig. 4C, V-2). The concepts of beam filtration and collimation are illustrated in Figure 5, V-2.

c. *Cone*. The long, open-ended, lead-lined cone used for dental x-ray machines reduces patient exposure compared to shorter cones or plastic pointed cones. Use of a long cone (16-in.) compared to shorter ones results in the use of a less divergent x-ray beam and, therefore, results in a smaller volume of patient tissues exposed. Lead-lined cones reduce the amount of scatter radiation at the end of the cone compared to non-lead-lined cones and, therefore, their use results in reduced patient exposure. Plastic pointed cones cause a significant increase in the amount of scatter radiation at the end of the cone and have been outlawed in several states for that reason. See Figure 6, V-2.

d. *Electronic timer*. The fast films currently used in dental radiography require the use of electronic

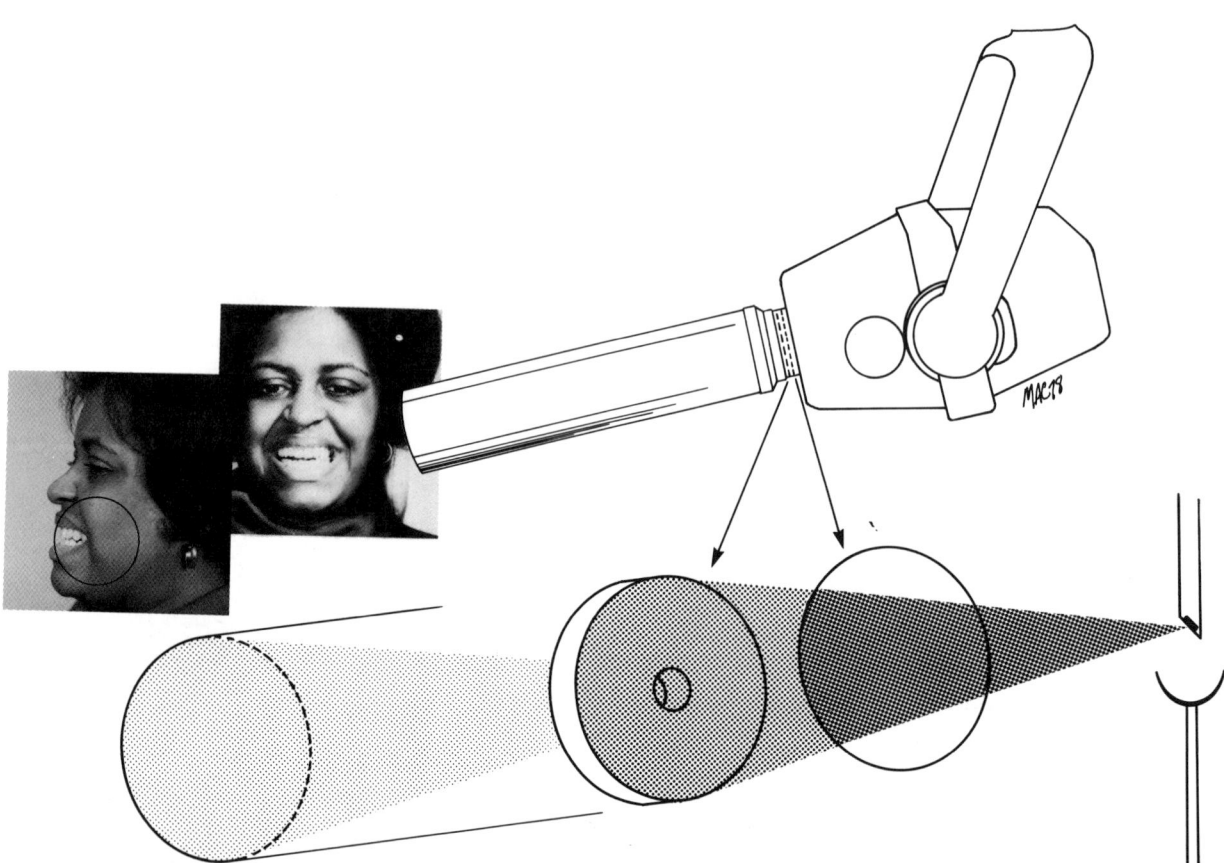

Fig. 5, V-2 Function of filter and collimator. Entire x-ray beam passes through the aluminum filter to remove the nonpenetrating, long-wavelength x rays. The collimator determines the size and shape of the useful beam.

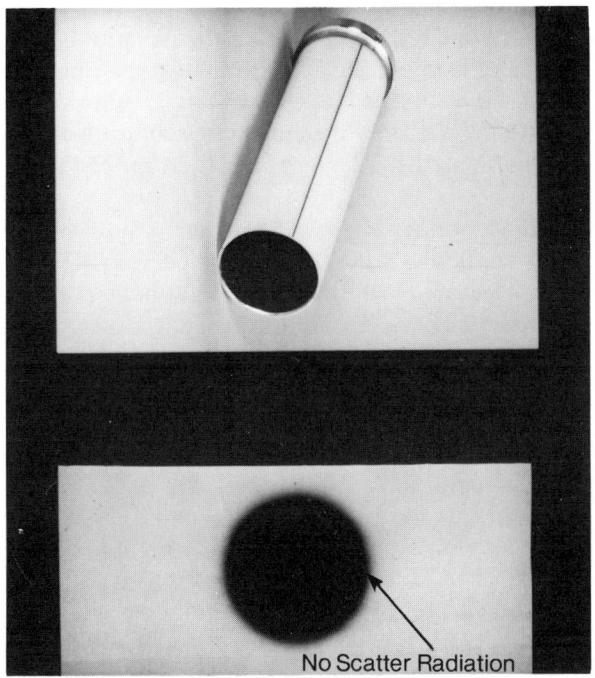

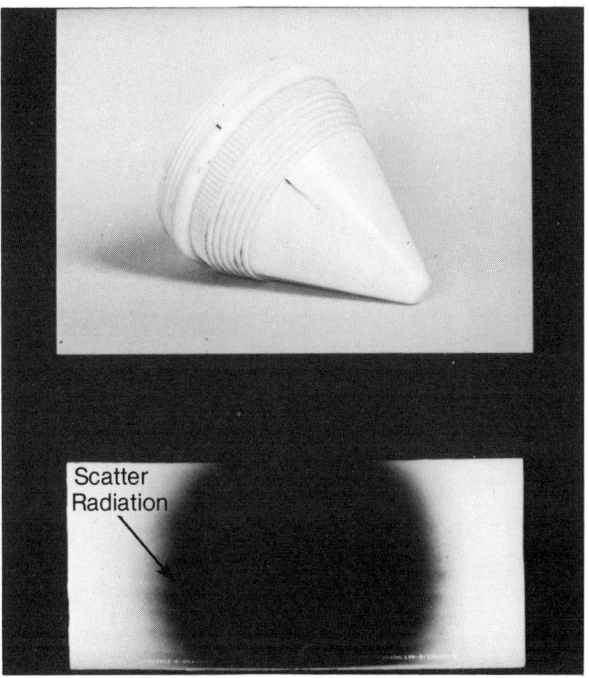

Fig. 6, V-2 A. Long, lead-lined cone with resulting x-ray beam.

B. Pointed plastic cone with resulting excess scatter radiation.

timers to accurately control the length of x-ray exposures. Previously, mechanical timers were used with slower films and were appropriate only for those slow films and, for this reason, mechanical timers are illegal in at least one state (North Carolina) (Fig. 7, V-2).

6. *High-speed film.* Ultraspeed (D speed) or Ektaspeed (E speed) films are recommended for intraoral radiography. Previously, slower-speed films (A, B, C) were used, and although the use of these films provided increased detail in the tooth images, the higher dose of x rays required was deemed unjustified to continue their use. Fast films are also available for panoramic and cephalometric radiography.

Operator Protection

All persons in the area in which radiographs are exposed are subject to exposure from both the primary beam and secondary radiation. Any person, operator, or other office staff member who is positioned in line with the x-ray cone may be exposed to relatively higher doses of radiation because the primary beam passes through the patient and travels some distance until absorbed by the air or some object. Secondary radiation is present throughout the operatory during the exposure. The procedure affording maximum operator protection is to position

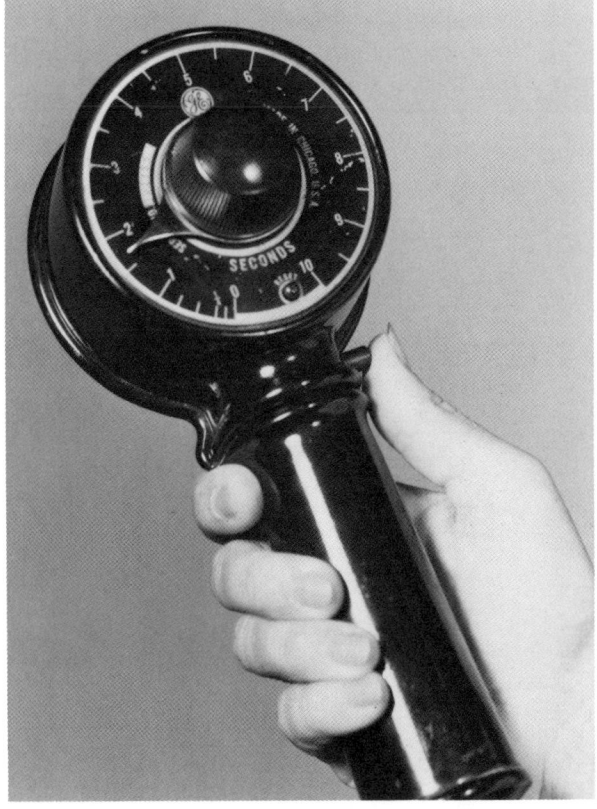

Fig. 7, V-2 An old outdated mechanical timer, *not* to be used with modern-day fast-speed film.

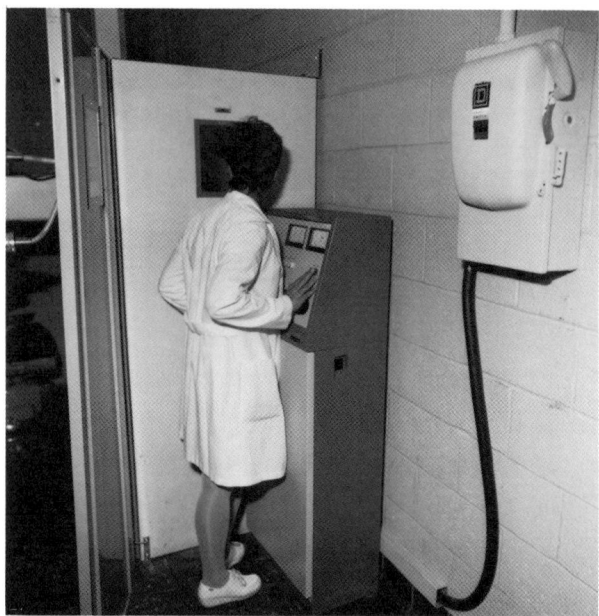

Fig. 8, V-2 Operator located behind lead barrier during exposure of radiographs.

the operator behind a protective barrier containing lead, thereby preventing all radiation, secondary or primary beam, from reaching the operator (Fig. 8, V-2). No other persons should be in the operatory, and consideration should be given to the composi-

tion of the walls if personnel such as the receptionist or laboratory technician are located in an adjacent room. If a lead barrier is not available, the operator should be positioned no closer than 6 feet from the patient and the x-ray machine and also in a location between 90 and 135 degrees from the x-ray cone (Fig. 9, V-2).

It is good radiographic practice to monitor and measure the radiation received by personnel working in the areas in which radiographs are taken. Commercially available film badge devices are worn during work hours, and a report is submitted by the film badge service, listing exposures received, if any (Fig. 10, V-2).

Radiation authorities have established exposure guidelines for persons, including dental personnel, who work in the vicinity of x-ray equipment. The *maximum permissible dose* (MPD) is thought to be that amount of *total body* radiation below which no harmful effects occur. No individual under age 18 is permitted to work as an x-ray operator, on the basis that growing and developing tissues are more susceptible to radiation injury. For persons over the age of 18, the accepted maximum permissible dose is 5 REM per year or 0.1 REM per week. (The value of a REM can be considered the same as a RAD.) These limits are established by the National Committee on Radiation Protection (NCRP). The formula for determining the maximum permissible dose is 5(N-18), where

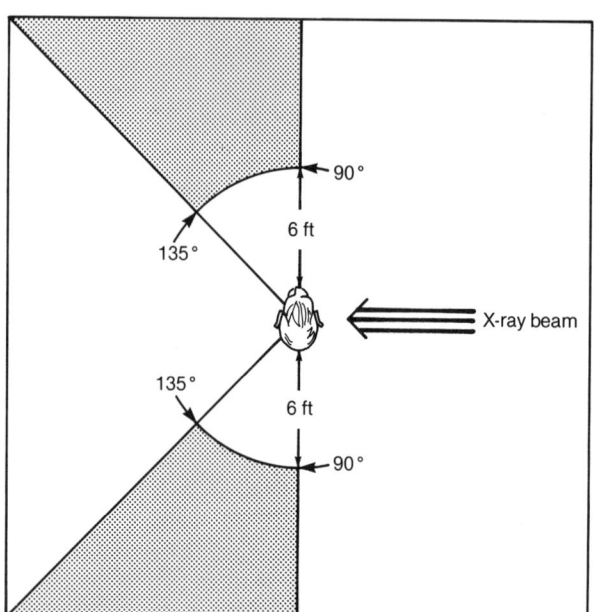

Fig. 9, V-2 Operator position if no lead barrier is available. Shaded areas represent positions of greatest safety. Minimum distance is 6 ft. behind the patient's

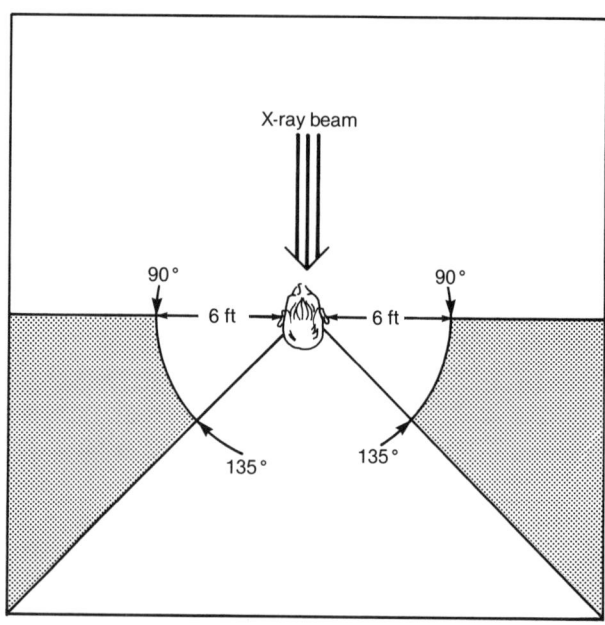

head. Location should be from 90–135 degrees from the x-ray cone.

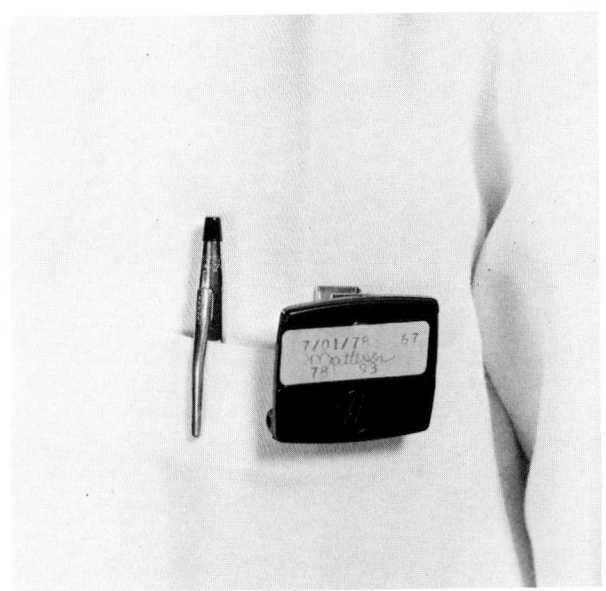

Fig. 10, V-2 Radiation monitoring badge.

BIBLIOGRAPHY

De Lyre, W. R., and Johnson, O. N. *Essentials of Dental Radiography for Dental Assistants and Hygienists.* 4th ed. Norwalk, Conn.: Appleton & Lange, 1990.

Frommer, H. H. *Radiology for Dental Auxiliaries.* 4th ed. St. Louis: C. V. Mosby Co., 1987.

Goaz, P. W., and White, S. C. *Oral Radiology: Principles and Interpretation.* 2d ed. St. Louis: C. V. Mosby Co., 1987.

N equals the age in years, which must be greater than 18. To calculate the maximum permissible dose for a 55-year-old individual:

$5(N-18)$ = Max. permissible dose (MPD)

$5(55-18)$ = MPD

$5 \times 37 = 185$ REM

The MPD is based on total body dose and not the exposure of a smaller portion of the body. Even though it is believed that no harmful effects are caused by x-ray exposure below this level, these authorities emphasize that the effects of low doses of x rays are not completely understood, and they recommend that all practical measures be employed to prevent any unnecessary exposure.

Section 2

Examination

In a few words, phrases, or sentences, answer the following questions. Use a separate sheet of paper.

1. What is ionization?
2. Why is ionization important in radiation biology?
3. What are genetic effects?
4. What are somatic effects?
5. How does the mechanism of indirect-radiation effects differ from direct effects?
6. List and describe four radiation effects on cells.
7. Which general categories of cells are more sensitive to radiation? Give three examples.
8. Which general categories of cells are less sensitive to radiation?
9. What is the basic mechanism of low-dose radiation damage to an organ?
10. How do radiation effects accumulate?
11. What two sites adjacent to the oral cavity are especially sensitive to radiation? What procedures can be followed to minimize radiation dose to these regions?
12. Define
    a. Roentgen
    b. RAD
    c. Primary beam
    d. Useful beam
    e. Secondary radiation
13. List six procedures used to reduce the patient's exposure to radiation.
14. Define: maximum permissible dose. What is the maximum permissible dose for a 30-year-old person?

Section 3

Radiographic Anatomy

The diagnosis of dental disease is made by detecting and identifying changes from the normal. The dental auxiliary must know normal radiographic anatomy to be able to critique film quality, to decide if films should be retaken, and to correctly place the films in film mounts. Normal radiographic anatomy seen in intraoral and panoramic radiographs is presented in this section.

OBJECTIVES

1. To correctly identify 21 maxillary landmarks using photographs of intraoral radiographs.
2. To correctly identify 11 mandibular landmarks using photographs of intraoral radiographs.
3. To correctly identify 10 anatomic landmarks and 5 artifacts using a photograph of a panoramic radiograph.
4. To correctly identify the primary and permanent teeth on panoramic radiographs of patients at ages 4, 8, and 11.

IMPORTANCE OF KNOWLEDGE OF NORMAL ANATOMY

A dentist determines a radiographic diagnosis on the basis of normal radiographic anatomy. A comparison is made between normal dental anatomy and the patient's abnormalities as seen on the radiograph.

It is also important for the radiographer to be able to recognize and identify normal radiographic anatomy. The anatomy seen on each film is used as a guide for the correct placement of the film packet in the mouth and analysis of the film quality. Before a correct diagnosis can be made, the dental auxiliary should evaluate the film for technical quality and decide if each film is of acceptable quality.

ANATOMIC LANDMARKS OF THE MAXILLARY ANTERIOR AREA

1. *Nasal fossa*: Air in the nasal cavities outlining the boundaries of the nasal walls.

2. *Nasal septum*: Thin midline bony wall separating the right and left nasal cavities.

3. *Floor of nasal cavity*: Bony walls forming the inferior boundary of the nasal fossae.

4. *Mid-palatine suture*: Radiolucent line along the center of the maxilla where the embryonic palatal shelves joined to form the palate.

5. *Anterior nasal spine*: V-shaped bony protuberance in midline extending forward from the inferior aspect of the nasal cavity to which is attached the nasal cartilage.

6. *Tooth*:

a. *Enamel*: Radiopaque cap covering the crown of the tooth.

b. *Dentin*: Hard structure of the tooth between the enamel and the pulp.

c. *Pulp*: Radiolucent area in the center of the root and crown representing soft tissue (nerves and blood supply).

7. *Incisive foramen*: Opening in palate posterior to the central incisor teeth through which pass the nasopalatine nerves and artery.

8. *Nose*: Soft tissue of the nose may be evident.

9. *Anterior extent of the maxillary sinus*: Radiolucent air in the maxillary sinus bounded by radiopaque wall extending forward over the canine region.

10. *Incisive fossa*: Indentation in the anterior surface of the maxilla between the roots of the lateral incisor and canine that may result in a radiolucent region on the film.

11. *Canine fossa*: Indentation in the anterior surface of the maxilla distal to the root of the canine that may result in a radiolucent area.

12. *Typical "Y" formation*: Radiopaque lines in Y shape formed by the intersection of the nasal floor and the anterior extent of the maxillary sinus.

See Figure 1, V-3.

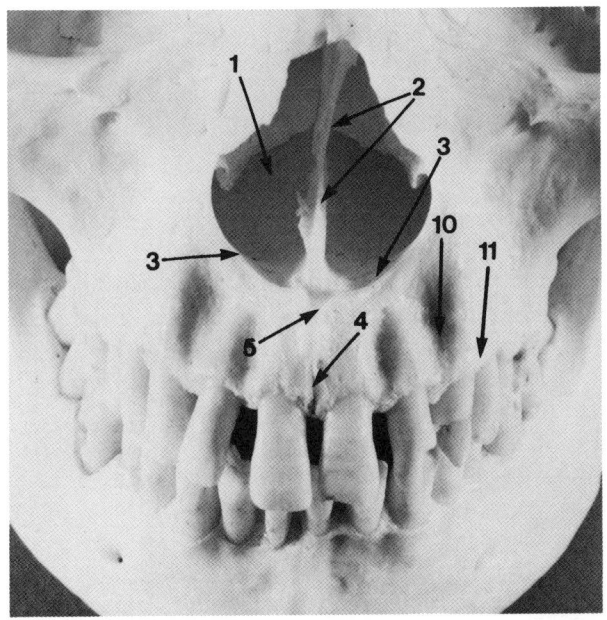

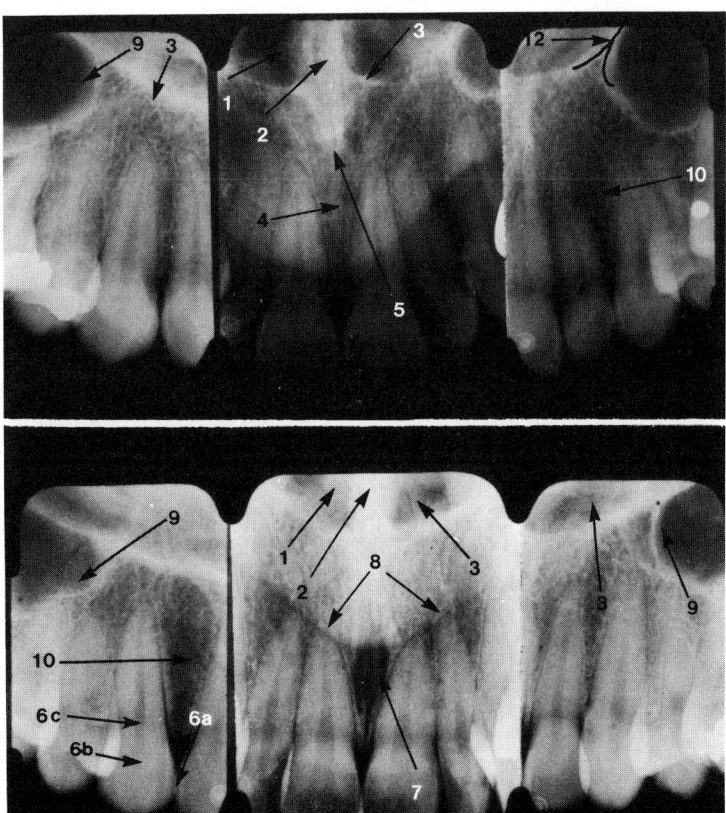

Fig. 1, V-3 Maxillary anterior area. Identify the listed anatomical sites using the numbers on the radiographs that correspond to the numbers in the list on the opposite page.

ANATOMIC LANDMARKS OF THE MAXILLARY POSTERIOR AREA

1. *Maxillary sinus*: Bilateral, radiolucent, air-filled cavities occupying a large portion of the maxilla above the posterior teeth.

2. *Inferior border of maxillary sinus*: Radiopaque line representing bony cortex of the inferior wall of the sinus.

3. *Zygomatic arch (malar process)*: Radiopaque bone located in the cheek joining with the maxilla, frontal, and temporal bones. The characteristic radiopaque "U" or "J" over the roots of the maxillary first or second molar represents the portion of the zygomatic arch that attaches to the maxilla.

4. *Maxillary tuberosity*: Curved bony eminence at distal end of maxillary alveolar ridges.

5. *Lateral pterygoid plate*: Thin, bony extension of the sphenoid bone to which are attached muscles of the throat and the lateral pterygoid muscle.

6. *Hamulus*: Bony spine extending downward from the medial pterygoid plate.

7. *Vessel in the wall of the maxillary sinus*: Radiolucent line representing a depression in the wall of the maxillary sinus for a vessel.

8. *Floor of nasal fossa*: Thin, radiopaque line along the top edge of maxillary posterior films representing the floor of the nasal fossa (or palate).

9. *Sinus septum*: Compartments formed within the maxillary sinus by bony walls which may be evident within the maxillary sinus.

10. *Coronoid process of mandible*: Thin, pyramid shape of the upper portion of the coronoid process of the mandible may be evident in maxillary molar projections.

See Figure 2, V-3

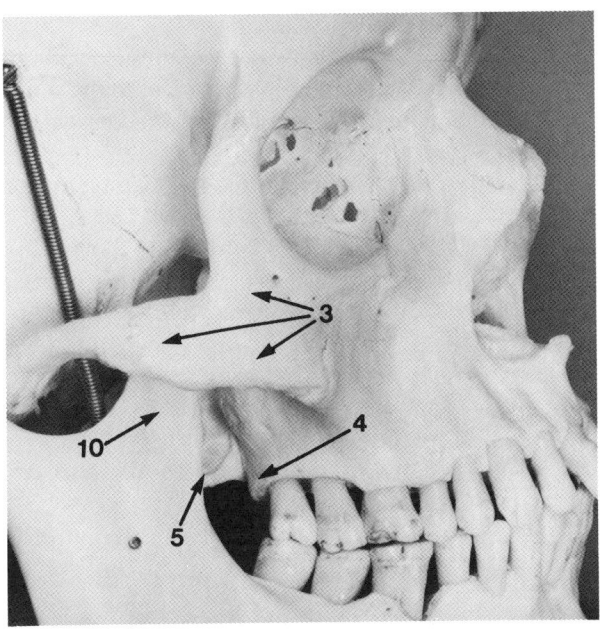

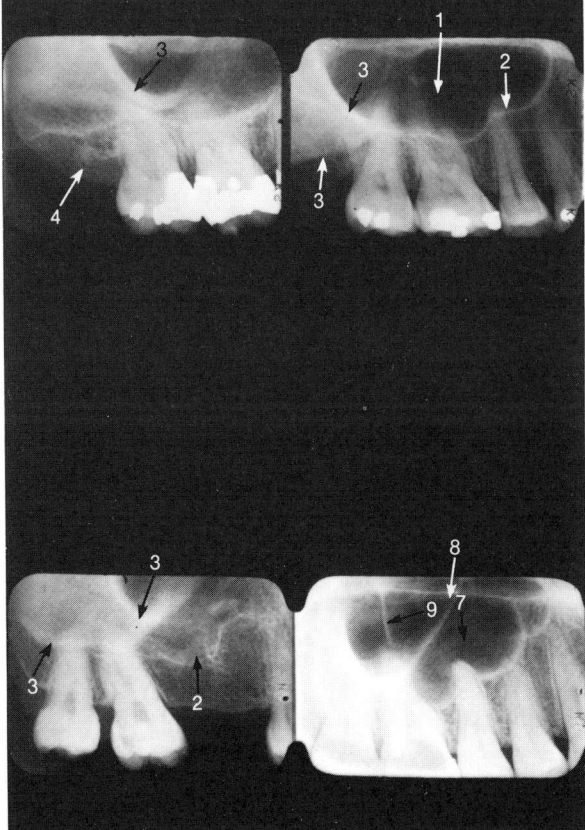
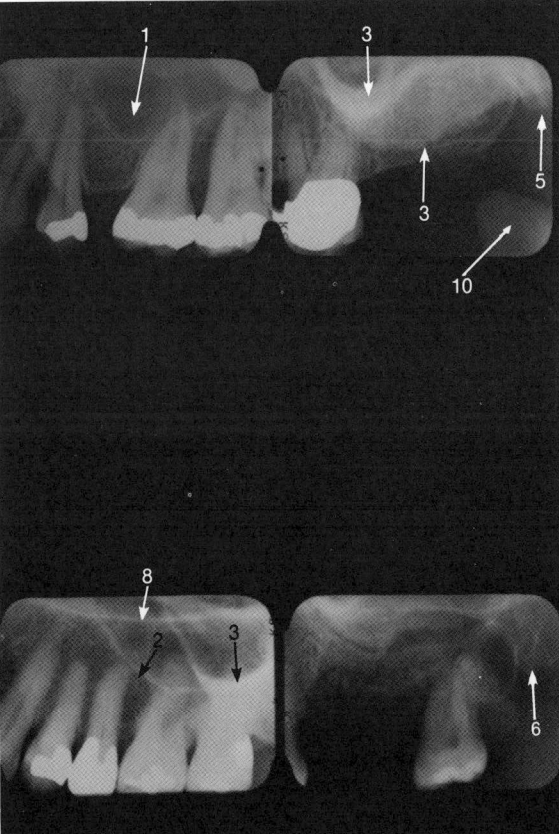

Fig. 2, V-3 Maxillary posterior area. Identify the listed anatomic sites using the numbers on the radiographs that correspond to the numbers in the list on the opposite page.

ANATOMIC LANDMARKS OF THE MANDIBULAR ANTERIOR AREA

1. *Inferior border of the mandible*: Thick radiopaque edge of the mandible.

2. *Genial tubercles*: Small bony spines located on the lingual side of the mandible adjacent to the midline for attachment of the geniohyoid and genioglossus muscles.

3. *Lingual foramen*: Small midline opening in lingual cortex of the mandible for a small vessel.

4. *Mental ridge*: Elevated bone along the anterior aspect of the mandible.

5. *Lip line*: The upper edge of the soft tissue lip may be evident.

6. *Nutrient canals*: Radiolucent grooves passing through alveolar bone representing vessels along the inner side of the bone cortex.

7. *Tori*: A bony prominence or protuberance on the lingual surface of the mandible.

See Figure 3, V-3.

Mandibular Anterior Area

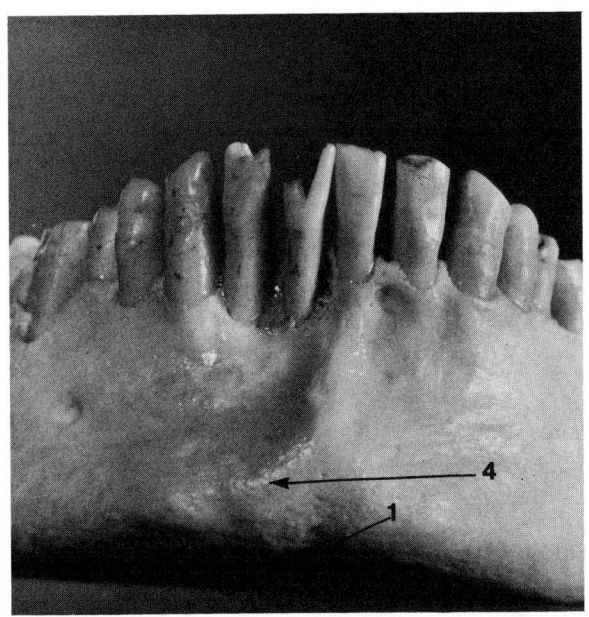

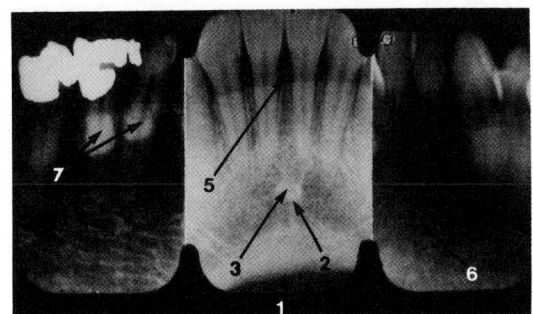

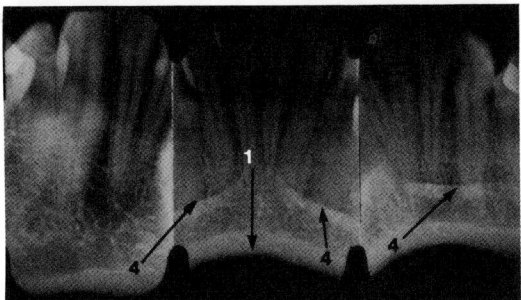

Fig. 3, V-3 Mandibular anterior area. Identify the listed anatomic sites using the numbers in the radiographs that correspond to the numbers in the list on the opposite page.

ANATOMIC LANDMARKS OF THE MANDIBULAR POSTERIOR AREA

1. *Mental foramen*: Radiolucent opening in facial side of mandible for the exit of the mental nerve.

2. *Mandibular canal*: Tube in the mandible extending from the mandibular foramen on the lingual side of the ramus, through the body of the mandible under the roots of the molar teeth, and ending at the mental foramen. The inferior alveolar nerve and artery pass through this canal.

3. *Internal oblique ridge (mylohyoid line)*: Ridge of bone extending along the lingual side of the mandible for the attachment of the mylohyoid muscle. This structure appears near the ends of the molar roots.

4. *Submandibular fossa*: Radiolucent area in the posterior body of the mandible below the internal oblique line representing a depression in the lingual side of the mandible for the submandibular salivary gland.

5. *External oblique line*: Radiopaque line along upper aspect of the posterior body of the mandible close to the necks of the molar teeth. The external oblique line is located on the facial side of the mandible and is the area into which the buccinator muscle attaches.

See Figure 4, V-3.

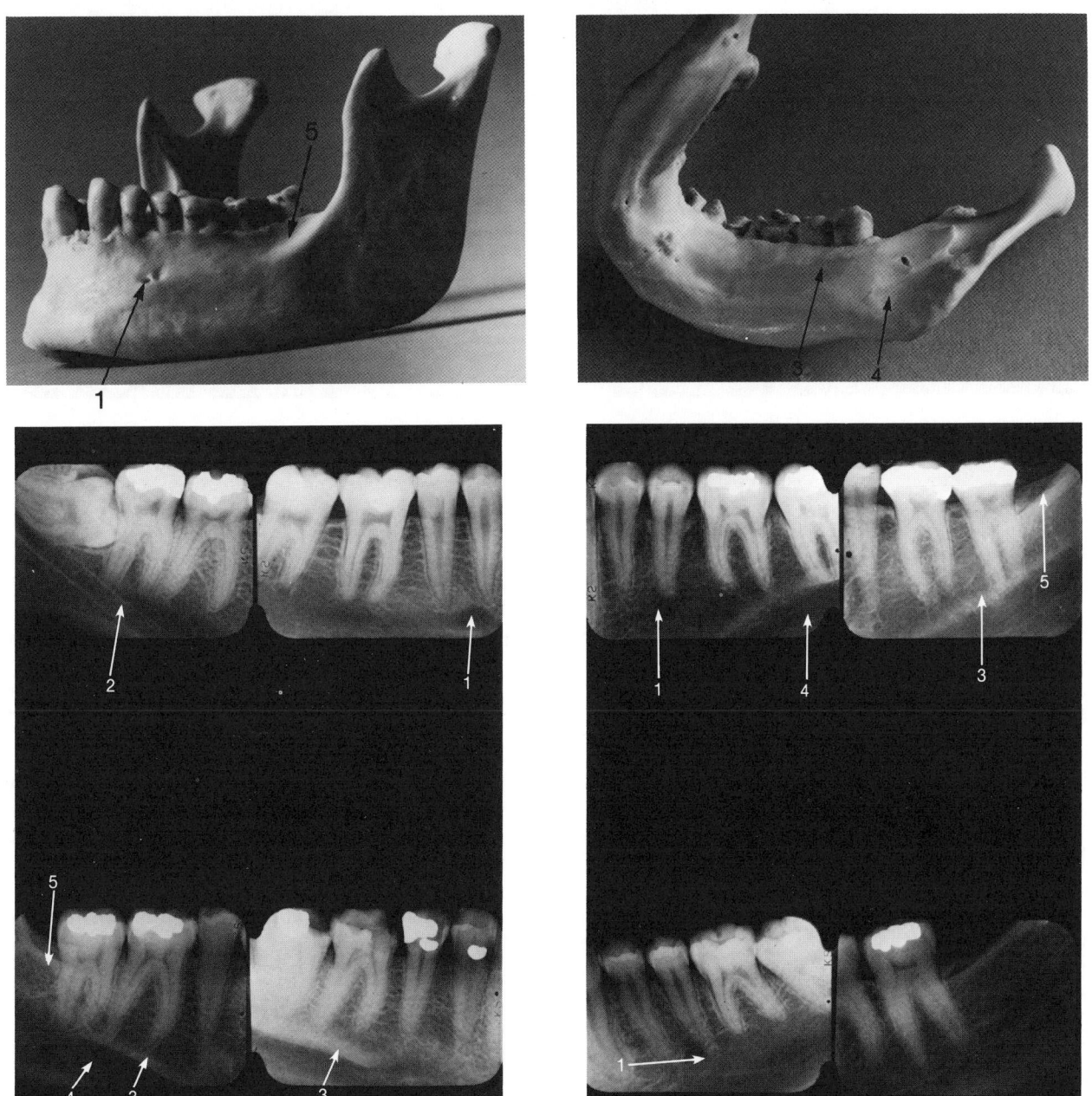

Fig. 4, V-3 Mandibular posterior area. Identify the listed anatomic sites using the numbers on the radiographs that correspond to the numbers in the list on the opposite page.

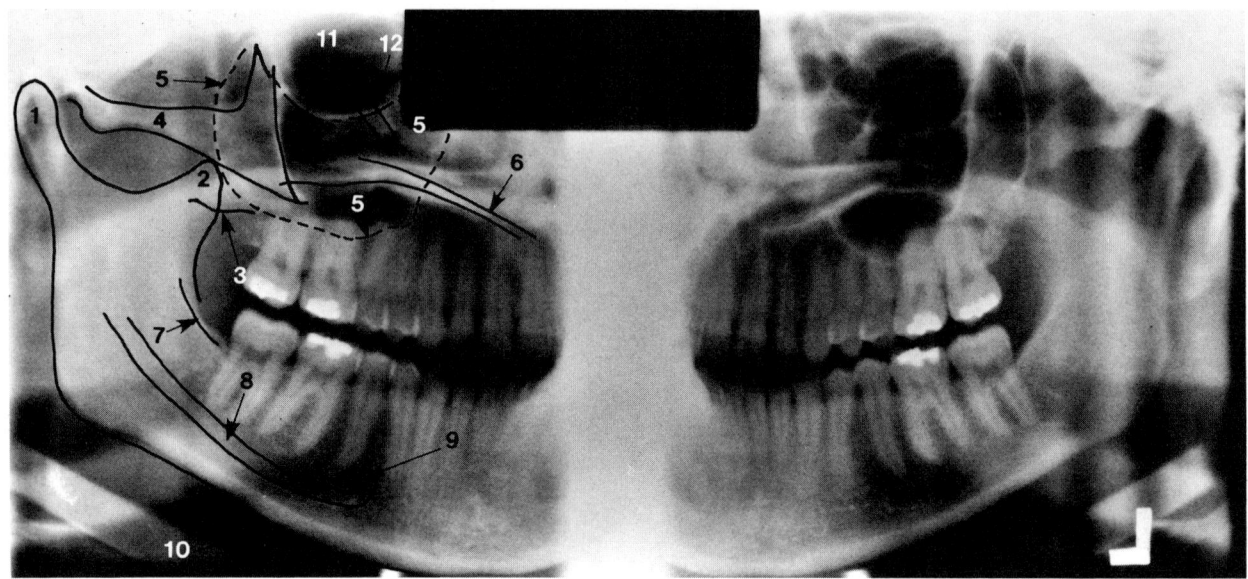

Fig. 5, V-3 Panoramic anatomy: (1) mandibular condyle, (2) coronoid process, (3) pterygoid plate, (4) zygomatic arch, (5) walls of maxillary sinus, (6) palate, (7) external oblique ridge, (8) mandibular canal, (9) mental foramen, (10) inferior border of the mandible, (11) orbital floor, and (12) infraorbital canal.

PANORAMIC ANATOMY

Panoramic radiographs are widely used in dentistry. With slightly less exposure than a full-mouth series of radiographs of periapicals and bitewings, the panoramic radiograph provides a broad overview of the entire dental arches and teeth on a 5-in. × 12-in. film. Figure 5, V-3 illustrates the radiographic anatomy shown on panoramic radiographs.

PANORAMIC ARTIFACTS

Even while following correct technique procedures, various artifacts are commonly present in panoramic films such as air spaces, soft-tissue shadows, and shadows from machine components (Fig. 6, V-3). These artifacts are superimposed over the bony landmarks on the panoramic x ray and should be recognized by the dental auxiliary to help evaluate the overall film quality.

ANATOMIC LANDMARKS OF CHILDREN

The growth and development of the teeth and jaws are coordinated and sequenced to provide a child with a primary set of 20 teeth that allows chewing during the early years. Later the increased jaw size allows for the development of the 32 larger permanent teeth. By about age 2 the 20 primary teeth are in place in the jaws while many of the permanent teeth are beginning to form beneath (Fig. 7A, V-3). Around age 6, the primary incisor teeth are lost and the permanent incisors erupt into position. The stage of development during which both primary and permanent teeth are erupted into chewing position is called the *mixed dentition* (Fig. 7B, V-3).

The final exchange of primary tooth loss and replacement with permanent successors occurs between ages 10 and 12. During this period the permanent canines and first and second premolars replace the primary canines and first and second primary molars (Fig. 7C, V-3).

BIBLIOGRAPHY

Berry, H. M. *Radiologic Anatomy of the Jaws*. Philadelphia: University of Pennsylvania Press, 1982.

Goaz, P. W., and White, S. C. *Oral Radiology: Principles and Interpretation*. 2d ed. St. Louis: C. V. Mosby Co., 1987.

Kasle, M. J. *An Atlas of Dental Radiographic Anatomy*. 3d ed. Philadelphia: W. B. Saunders Co., 1989.

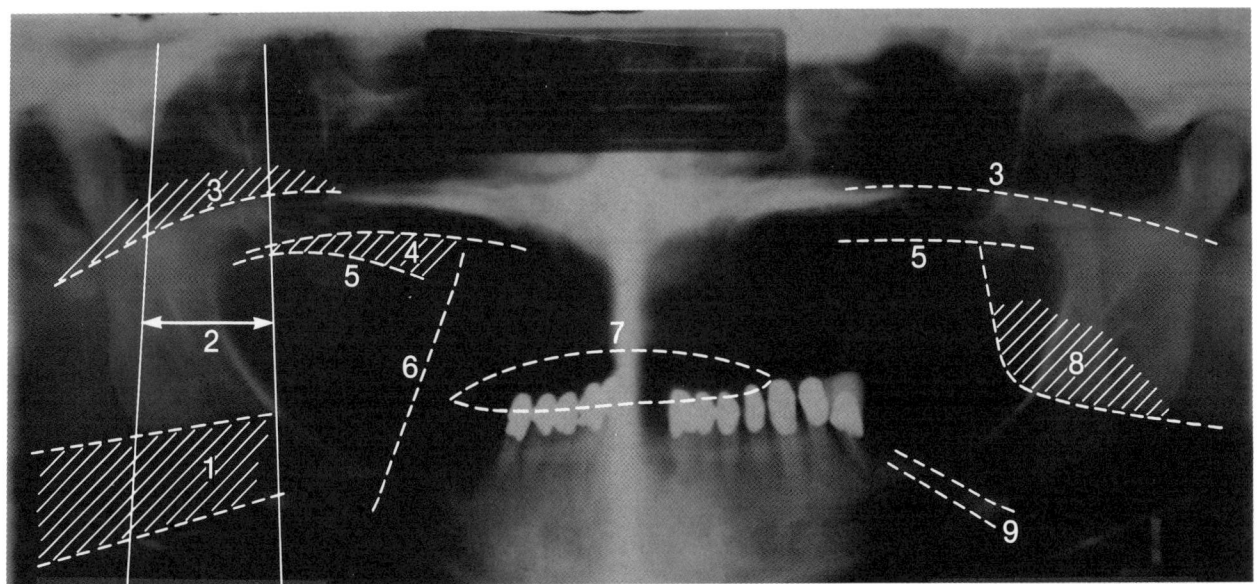

Fig. 6, V-3 Panoramic artifacts: (1) soft tissue shadow, (2) pancentric head positioning device, (3) nasal airway shadow, (4) oral airway shadow, (5) top of tongue line, (6) nasolabial fold, (7) lip line, (8) ghost shadow of opposite mandible, and (9) ghost shadow of opposite chin rest.

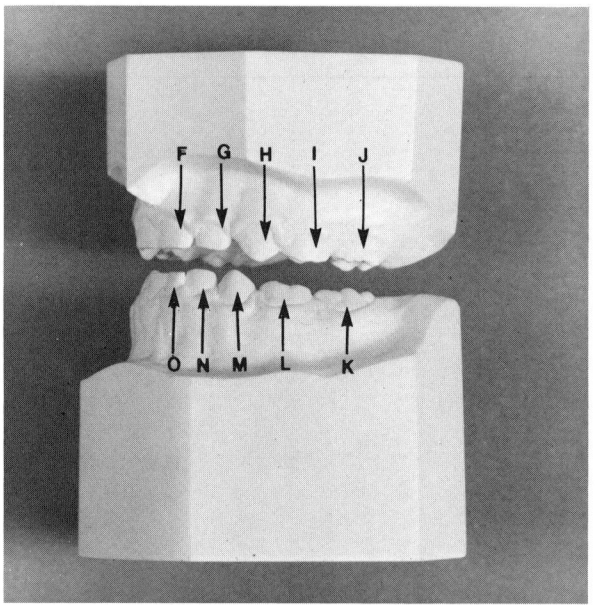

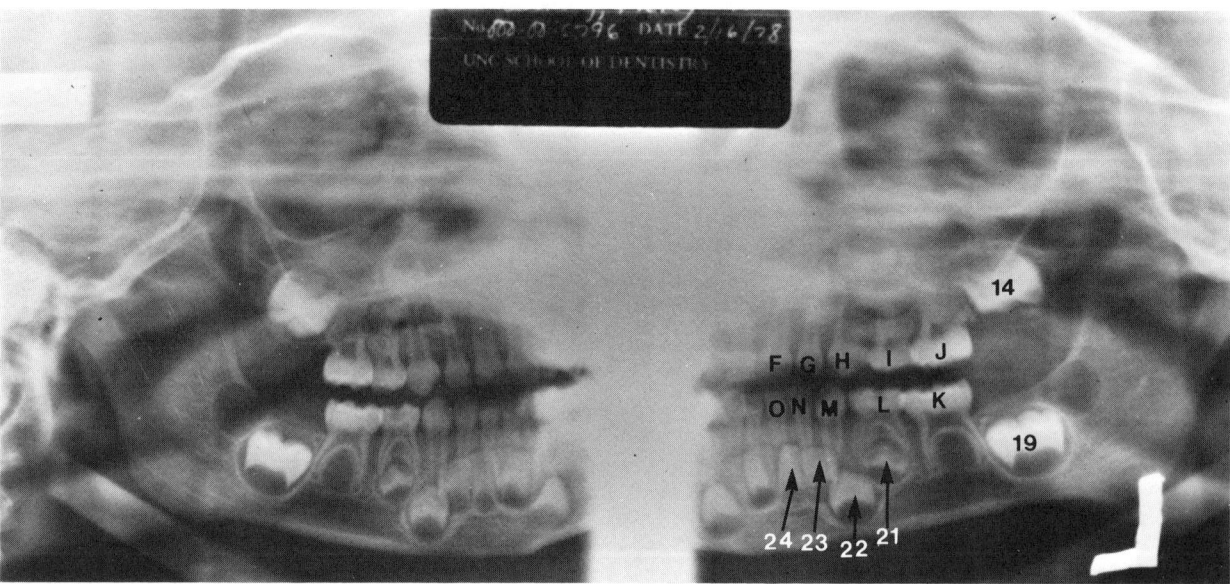

Fig. 7, V-3 A. Radiographic anatomy, 4-year-old patient. Identify the primary and permanent teeth on the study models and panoramic radiographs. The anterior region is shown twice on this type of panoramic film. Numbers signify permanent teeth and letters indicate primary teeth.

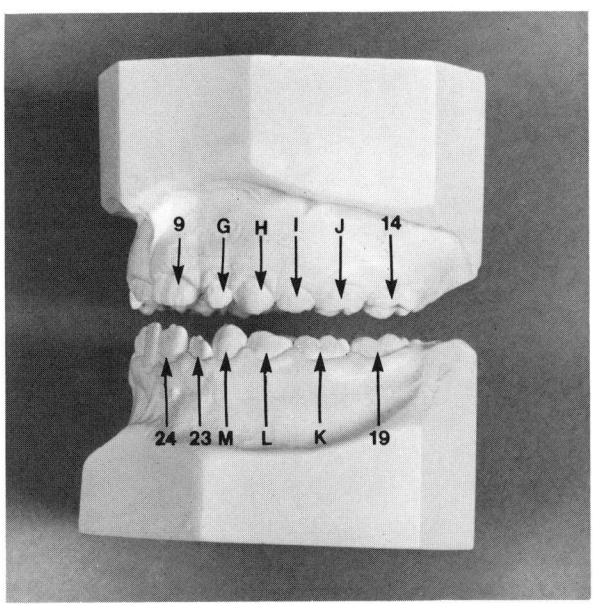

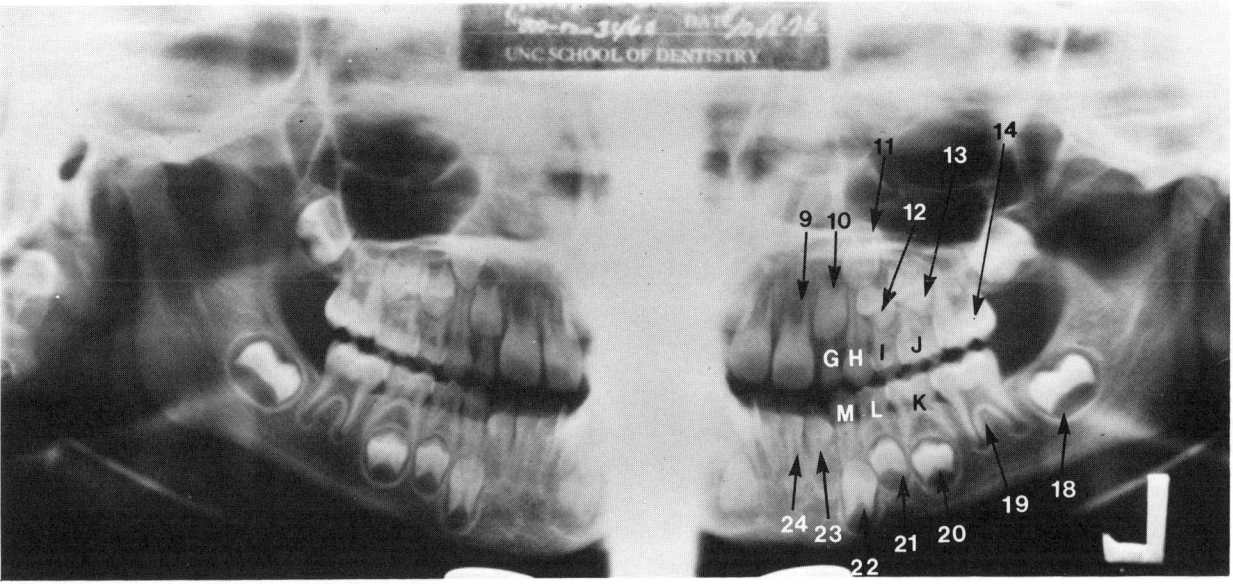

B. Radiographic anatomy, 8-year-old patient.

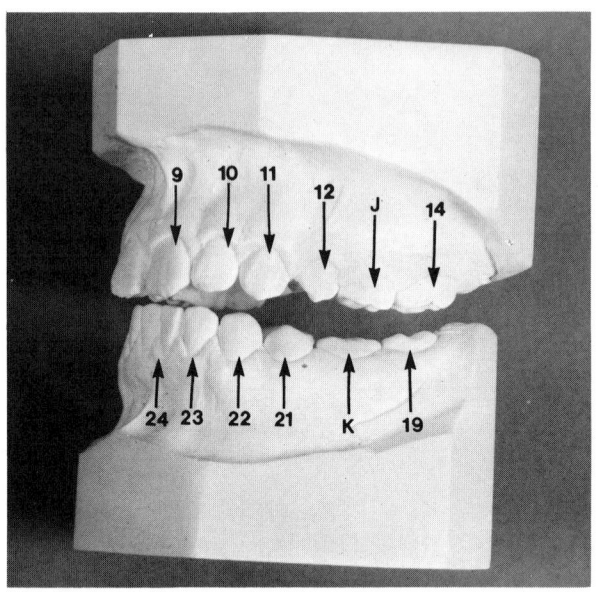

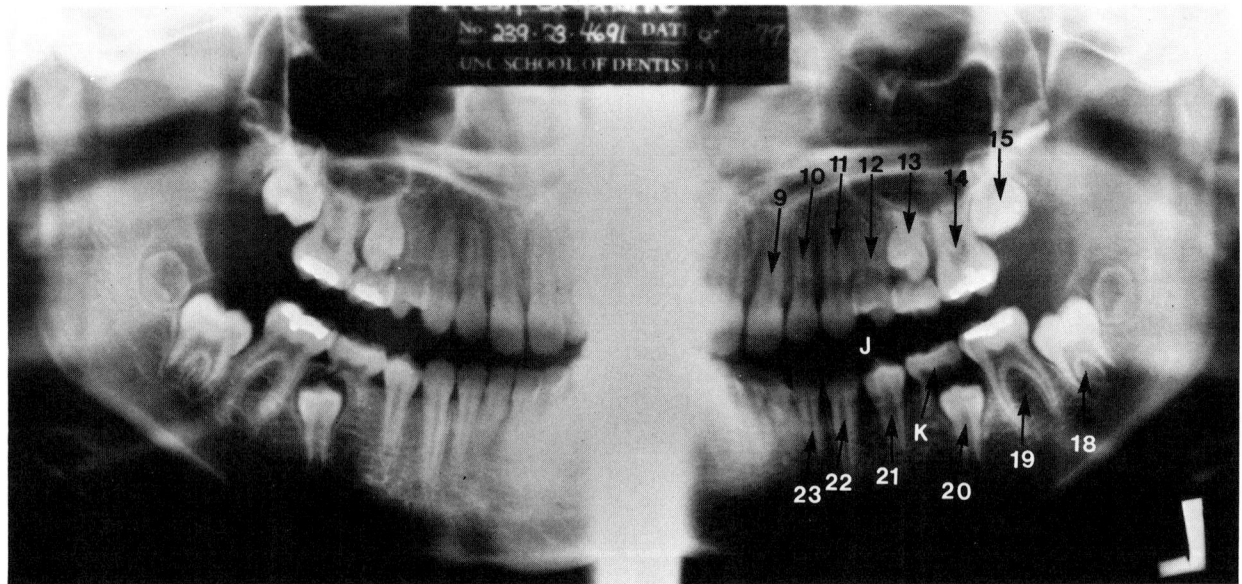

C. Radiographic anatomy, 11-year-old patient.

Section 3

Examination

I. List the maxillary landmarks labeled in Figures 1, 2, and 3 in the spaces below.

1. _____

2. _____

3. _____

4. _____

5. _____

6. _____

7. _____

8. _____

9. _____

10. _____

11. _____

12. _____

13. _____

14. _____

15. _____

16. _____

17. _____

18. _____

19. _____

20. _____

21. _____

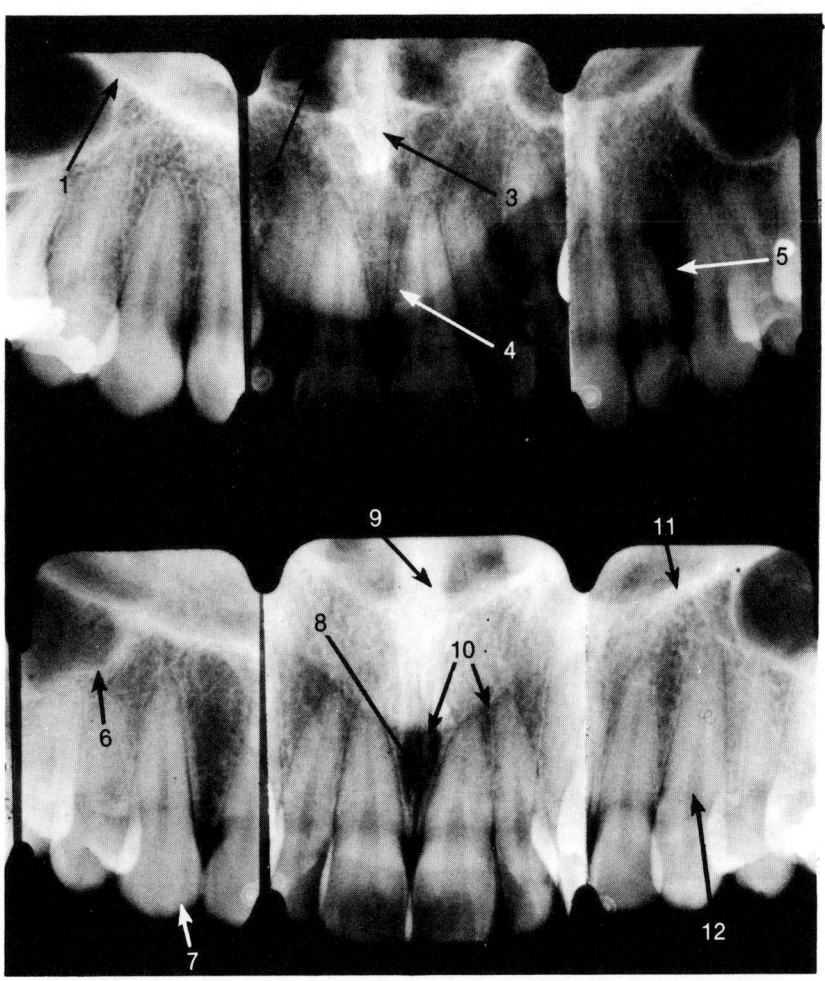

Fig. 1

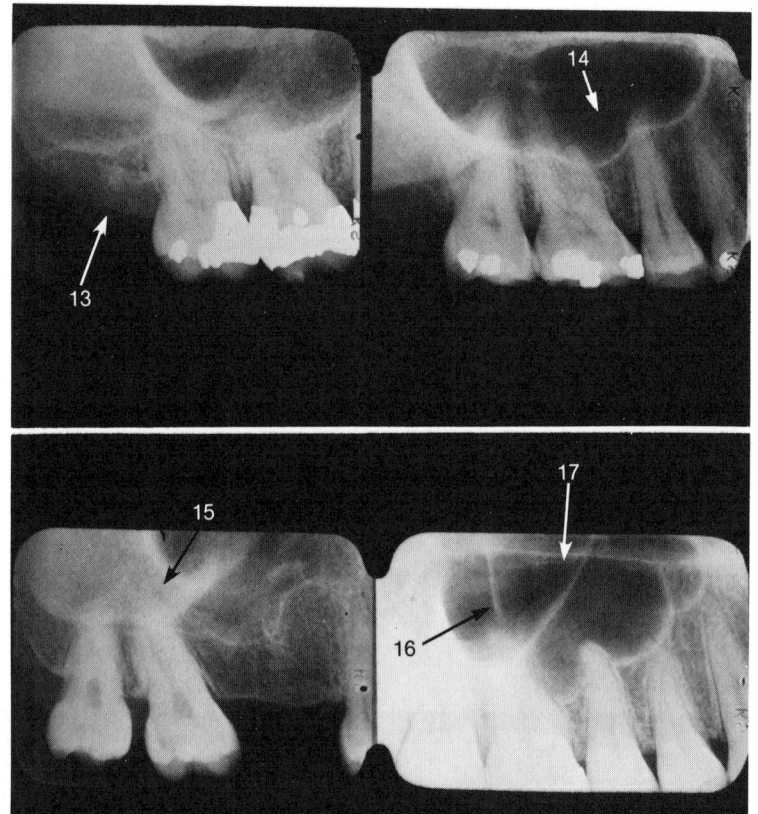

Fig. 2

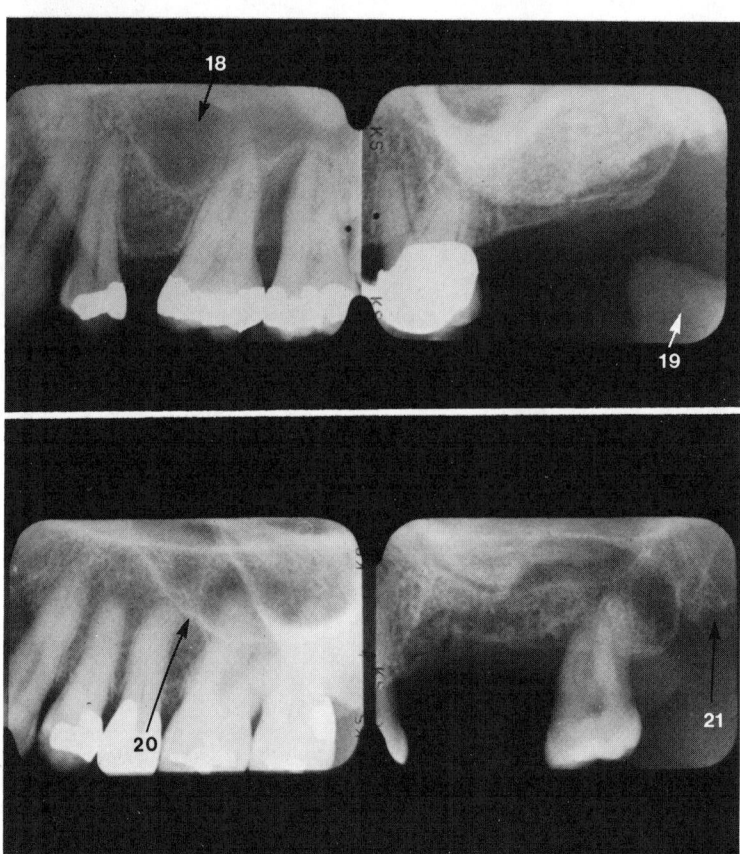

Fig. 3

46

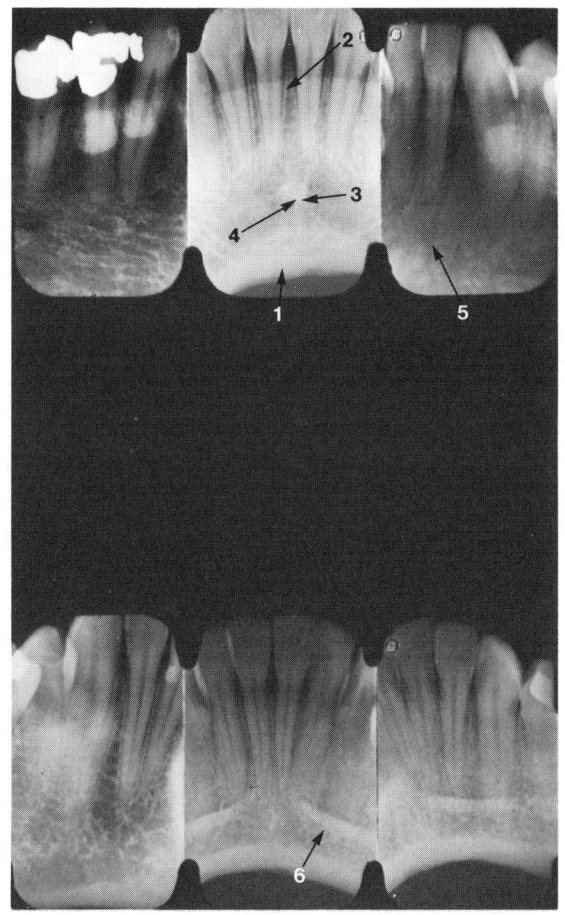

Fig. 4

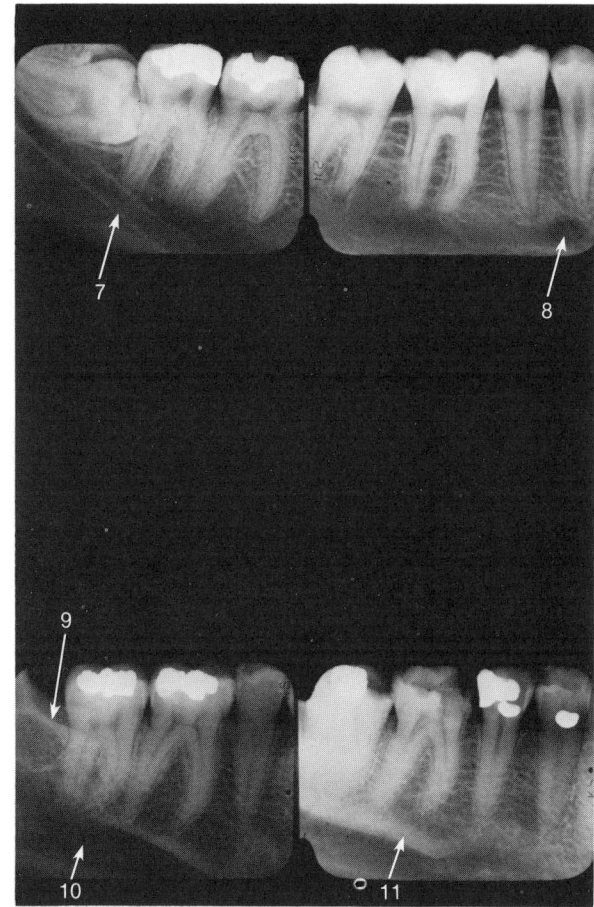

Fig. 5

II. List the mandibular landmarks labeled in Figures 4 and 5 in the spaces below.

1. _____

2. _____

3. _____

4. _____

5. _____

6. _____

7. _____

8. _____

9. _____

10. _____

11. _____

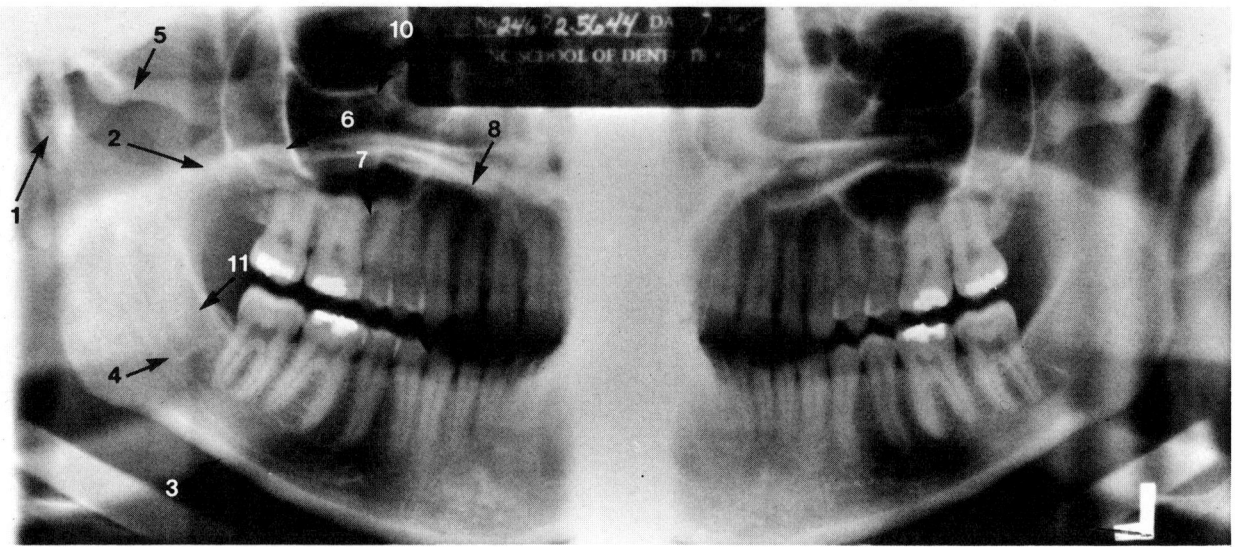

Fig. 6

III. Identify the landmarks in the labeled panorex radiograph in Figure 6 in the spaces below.

1. _____

2. _____

3. _____

4. _____

5. _____

6. _____

7. _____

8. _____

9. _____

10. _____

11. _____

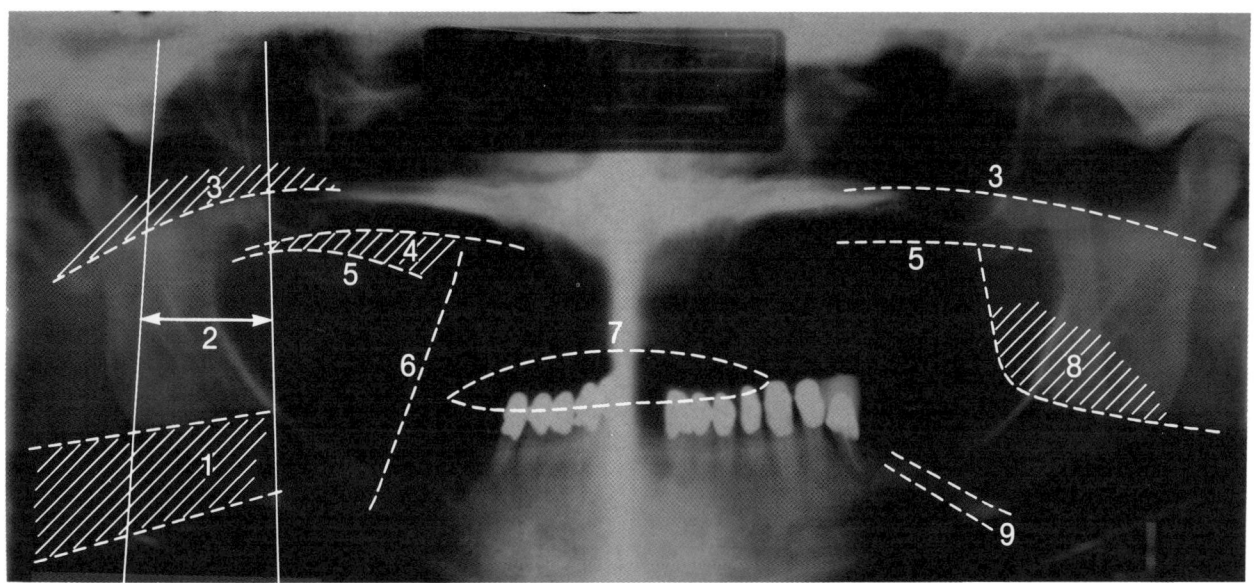

Fig. 7

IV. Identify artifacts in the labeled panoramic radiograph in Figure 7 in the spaces below.

1. _____

2. _____

3. _____

4. _____

5. _____

6. _____

7. _____

8. _____

9. _____

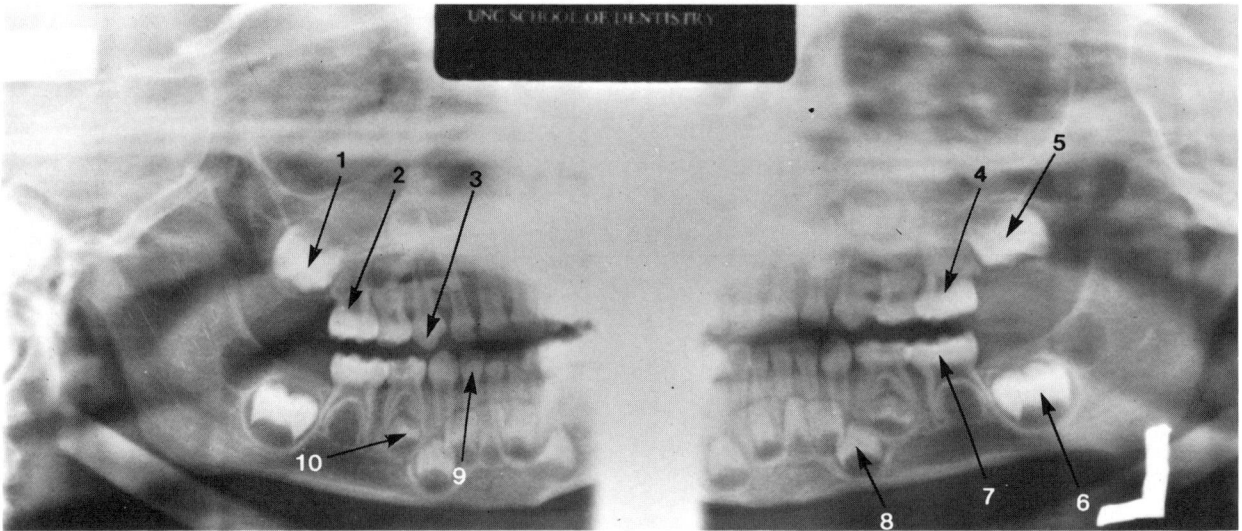

Fig. 8

V. Identify the teeth labeled in the panorex radiograph in Figure 8 in the spaces below.

1. _____

2. _____

3. _____

4. _____

5. _____

6. _____

7. _____

8. _____

9. _____

10. _____

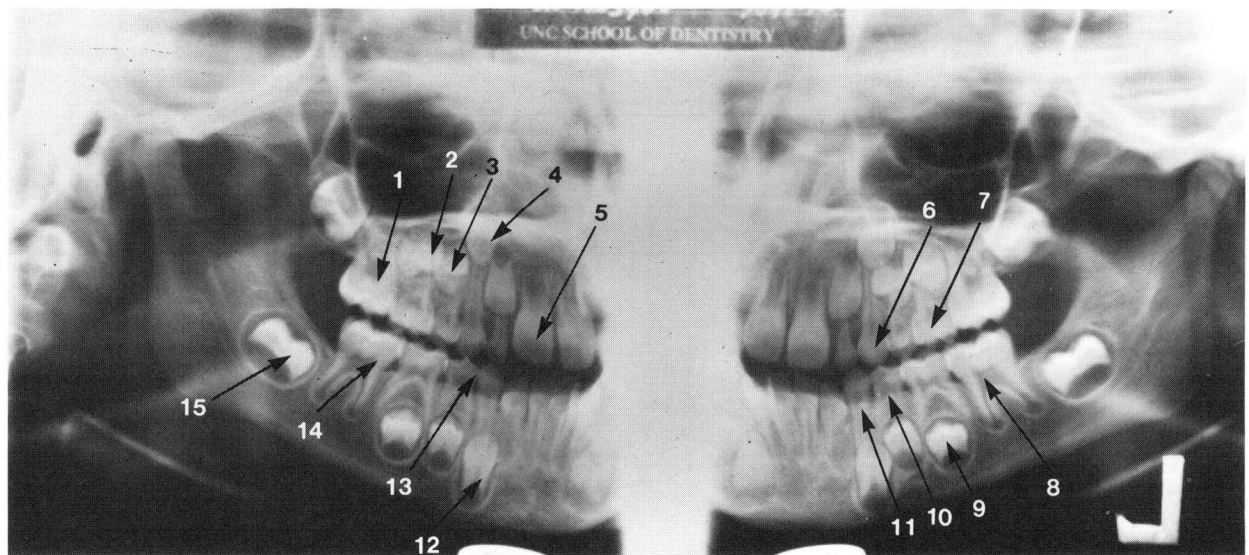

Fig. 9

VI. Identify the teeth labeled in the panorex radiograph in Figure 9 in the spaces below.

1. _____

2. _____

3. _____

4. _____

5. _____

6. _____

7. _____

8. _____

9. _____

10. _____

11. _____

12. _____

13. _____

14. _____

15. _____

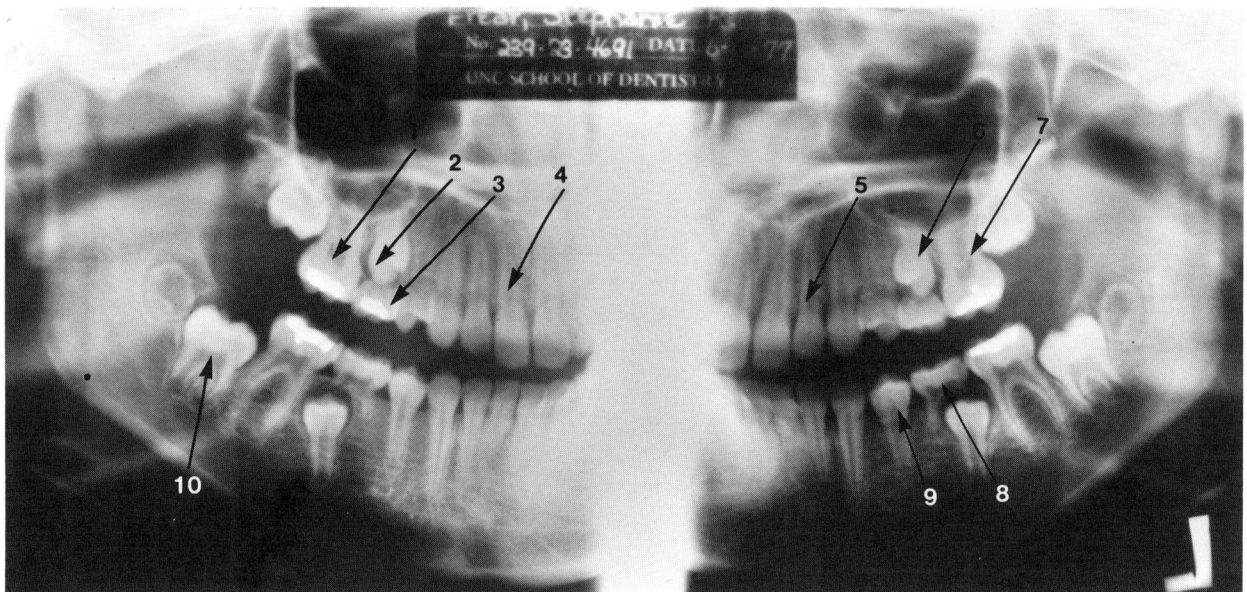

Fig. 10

VII. Identify the teeth labeled in the panorex radiograph in Figure 10 in the spaces below.

1. _____

2. _____

3. _____

4. _____

5. _____

6. _____

7. _____

8. _____

9. _____

10. _____

Section 4

The Film and the Darkroom

Knowledge of radiographic film, image formation, darkroom design, and processing procedures ensures that
optimum radiographic images are produced.

OBJECTIVES

1. To list the two basic components of radiographic film and to describe their composition.
2. To describe the factors that determine the
speed of the film.
3. To define and compare "screen" and "non-
screen" film.
4. To describe the types of film used in the
dental office.
5. To discuss the events that take place in the
film emulsion during the exposure and
processing of the film.
6. To define density, contrast, and detail.
7. To discuss four requirements for the design of
a dental darkroom.
8. To list the two types of lights used in a darkroom and to describe the use and components of a safelight.
9. To list two methods used to test a darkroom
for light leaks.
10. To describe the parts and use of a developing
tank.
11. To discuss the method used to maintain the
temperature of the processing chemicals.
12. To list the advantages of automatic processors
and to give the method used to process film
quickly.
13. To list three darkroom accessories and to
describe their functions.
14. To list and give the action of the components
of the developer and fixer.
15. To list procedures for darkroom upkeep.
16. To identify the principles of "quality assurance" in dental radiography.
17. To list the advantages of automatic processors.
18. To describe the time-temperature processing
method.
19. To list the steps used to process films in the
wet-tank system.
20. To describe film mounting procedures.

THE FILM

The radiographic film is an important tool that
is used by the dentist for diagnostic purposes. When
a radiograph is taken, certain images are produced
on the film that indicate anatomical shapes and tissue densities present in the oral cavity. The process
of film construction incorporates into the film certain
inherent characteristics that enable the film to produce these images. There are many types and uses of
x-ray films, and it is the responsibility of the radiographer to select the correct type of film and to utilize
it according to the specifications of the manufacturer.

FILM COMPOSITION

All radiographic film has two basic components:
the base and the emulsion. The *base* is a clear plastic
(cellulose acetate) with a slightly bluish tint to en-
hance image quality. Its primary function is to serve
as a stable support for the radiographic emulsion.
The base, which has a thickness of 0.007 in., provides
strength to the film and permits easy handling during processing and viewing procedures. It is also
constructed to withstand variations in heat, moisture, and chemicals during film processing.

The *emulsion* is a coating on the base and is firmly attached by a thin layer of adhesive. The adhesive
ensures a uniform distribution of emulsion over the
base, which contributes to sharp and distinct images

on the film. Applying the emulsion is the final procedure in film construction, and the green finish one sees upon opening a piece of x-ray film to light is due to the emulsion.

The radiographic emulsion is made of gelatin and silver bromide. The primary function of the gelatin is to suspend the silver bromide crystals over the film base so that they are evenly distributed. The silver bromide crystals are that part of the emulsion that is changed by the rays as they pass through the film.

FILM SPEED

The speed and/or sensitivity of radiographic film refers to the amount or quantity of x radiation required to change the state of the silver bromide crystals into a latent image. The film sensitivity is determined during production by controlling the concentration of crystals in the emulsion as well as the temperature under which they are added to the gelatin. During this process, crystals of varying sensitivity are produced. How sensitive they become is determined by the crystal size as well as its structural perfection; generally the larger crystals produce a faster film.

By regulating the size of the crystals, the manufacturer increases or decreases the film speed. These variations affect not only the sharpness of the image, but determine the amount of x-ray exposure (mA, time, kVp) needed to expose the film. Faster film means less exposure to x radiation for the patient but results in an image that is not as clearly defined. The reason is that the crystals are larger and appear more grainy on the film, and these images are said to have less resolution. Slower film is made up of smaller crystals that produce images with greater detail; however, exposure to x radiation is longer. These films are said to have greater definition and resolution.

TYPES OF FILM

There are two basic types of film: "nonscreen" and "screen." Nonscreen film is available in speeds identified by letters ranging from "A" to "F" with "A" referring to the slowest and "F" indicating the fastest. Due to larger patient exposure doses on film types "A," "B," and "C," only "D" and "E" speed films are recommended for intraoral use. "E" speed film can be exposed approximately twice as fast as "D" speed

film; therefore, it delivers about one-half the amount of radiation to the patient. There is a decrease in image quality as the film speed increases, but there are indications that the "D" and "E" films are of equal usefulness in dental radiography. The "F" speed designation has been reserved for a faster emulsion that could be produced in the future.

FILM INVENTORY

The responsibility for maintaining x-ray film supply is usually assigned to the dental radiographer. The radiographer must monitor film use to be sure that an adequate supply is available to meet the radiographic demands of the dental practice. X-ray film has a limited shelf life, although this may be extended slightly through refrigeration. It is important to maintain fresh film supplies, so the radiographic film packages are provided with expiration dates by the manufacturer (Fig. 1, V-4). As a rule, an order for film should be placed when two to three weeks supply of film remains in stock. This should allow sufficient time for fresh film to arrive.

SCREEN FILM AND EXTRAORAL PROJECTIONS

Extraoral projections refer to radiographic procedures in which the x-ray film remains outside the patient's mouth during the exposure and screen-type film is utilized. This type of examination incorporates the use of a light-free film-holding device, a cassette, into which the screen film is placed prior to exposure (Fig. 2, V-4). Inside the covers of the cassette, intensifying screens are installed which are made of calcium

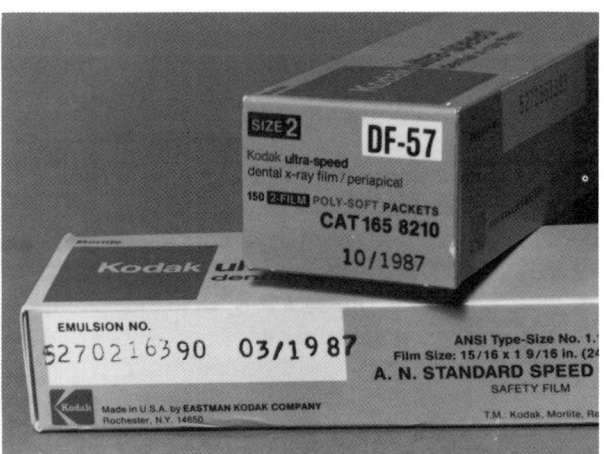

Fig. 1, V-4 Dated film boxes help ensure a fresh film inventory.

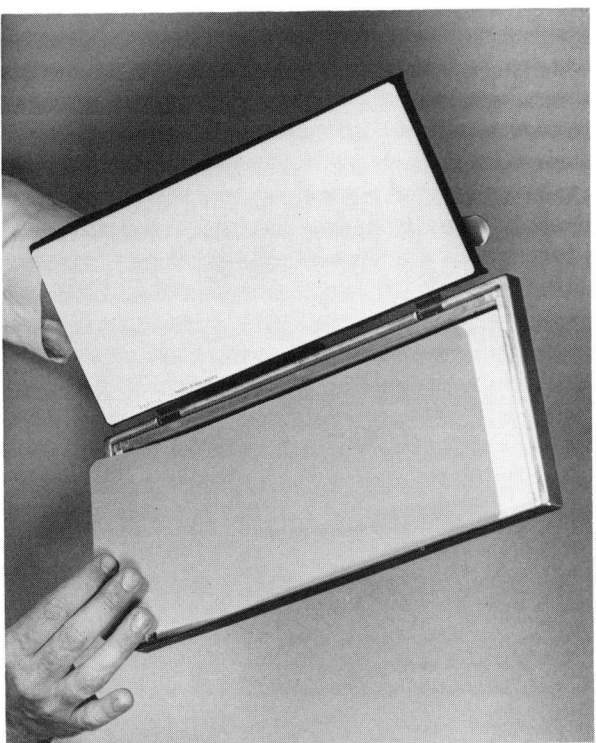

Fig. 2, V-4 Cassette with film.

tungstate coated on a film base. The screens are cut according to the size of the cassette and are smooth, allowing the film to be placed firmly against their surfaces, thus ensuring close screen-film contact during the exposure. Film is purchased in sizes to match the cassette being utilized. Cassettes, screens, and film are available in a variety of sizes, accommodating a variety of procedures.

Routine extraoral procedures in the dental office are panoramic and cephalometric films. The lateral oblique view of the mandible is also done occasionally. The advantage of a screen film system is that a larger or more dense area can be radiographed using less x-ray exposure. The screens inside the cassette are able to convert small amounts of x-ray energy into a green or blue-violet light, which in turn exposes the screen film inside the cassette. It should be noted that screen film is manufactured to be extremely sensitive to light of the green or blue-violet spectrum. When the cassette is exposed to radiation, light is emitted by the intensifying screens. The major portion of exposure of the film is due to the light emission rather than to x rays hitting the film. Although there is loss in the definition of the images, the films are adequate for many purposes and the patient is exposed to much less radiation.

NONSCREEN FILM AND INTRAORAL PROJECTIONS

The intraoral film fits inside the mouth, and the images result from direct exposure to x rays because no intensifying screens are used. Dental diagnosis requires fine detail in the films, and the use of nonscreen film is the only way to obtain the required information. Each film is packaged individually in light-tight, moisture-resistant, flexible packets that are suitable for intraoral use. They are available in a variety of sizes to accommodate different needs and patient sizes.

Each film packet contains one or two pieces of x-ray film, two pieces of black protective paper, and lead-foil backing to absorb back-scatter radiation and to prevent it from reaching the film. Plastic or paper wrapping surrounds the content of the film packet to prevent saliva from reaching the film once it has been placed inside the oral cavity (Fig. 3, V-4). The packaging also protects the film from accidental exposure to white light. Film sizes are labeled as follows: #0, the smallest size available, used for child patients; #1, used most often for anterior periapical projections; #2, used for both adult periapical and bitewing films; and #3, occlusal film and is used as survey film. All of these films are used for multiple purposes, depending on patient size and the specific diagnostic requirements (Fig. 4, V-4).

FORMATION OF THE LATENT IMAGE

A latent image refers to the changes that occur in the film emulsion as a result of x-ray exposure. These changes are not visible to the eye and cannot be seen until the film is processed. The latent image occurs when the x rays pass through the emulsion and cause changes in the sensitive silver bromide crystals. The image one sees when viewing radiographs is the transformation of the sensitized silver bromide into blackened metallic silver. See Figure 5, V-5.

CHARACTERISTICS OF OPTIMUM IMAGE

Density refers to the blackening effect or darkness that occurs on the film when it is exposed to radiation and then processed. The density of the film image is seen when the film is placed on the viewbox and is radiolucent or radiopaque in different areas. Radiolucent areas indicate that the x-ray beam

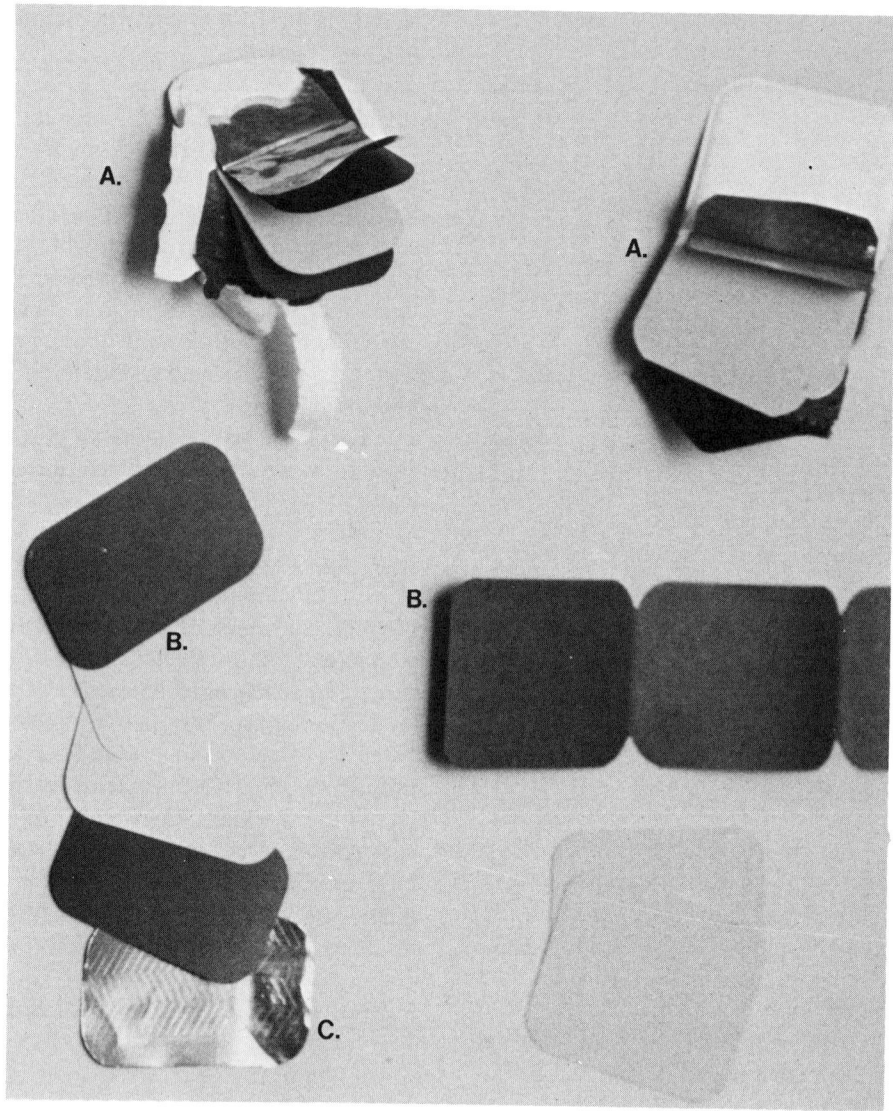

Fig. 3, V-4 Contents of periapical packet. A. Periapical packets opened.
B. Black paper. C. Lead foil.

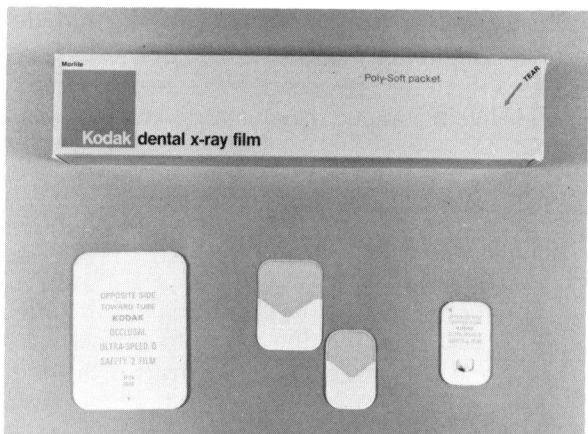

Fig. 4, V-4 Packet sizes. Intraoral packets are available in different sizes.

passed through less dense tissue such as sinuses, a foramen, or soft tissues such as the lip. For radiopaque areas, the reverse is true. Light areas on the film indicate that the x-ray beam was absorbed by the thickness and density of tissues (such as teeth and bones), and that the rays never reached and exposed the film.

Interpretation of the radiograph for diagnosis purposes requires the viewer to have an understanding of these densities, what they represent, and whether they have normal anatomical appearances. The radiographer's responsibility is to be able to produce radiographs of proper density, which are free of artifacts and have clearly defined structural edges that allow for correct interpretation of the patient's dental condition. A major task of the radiographer

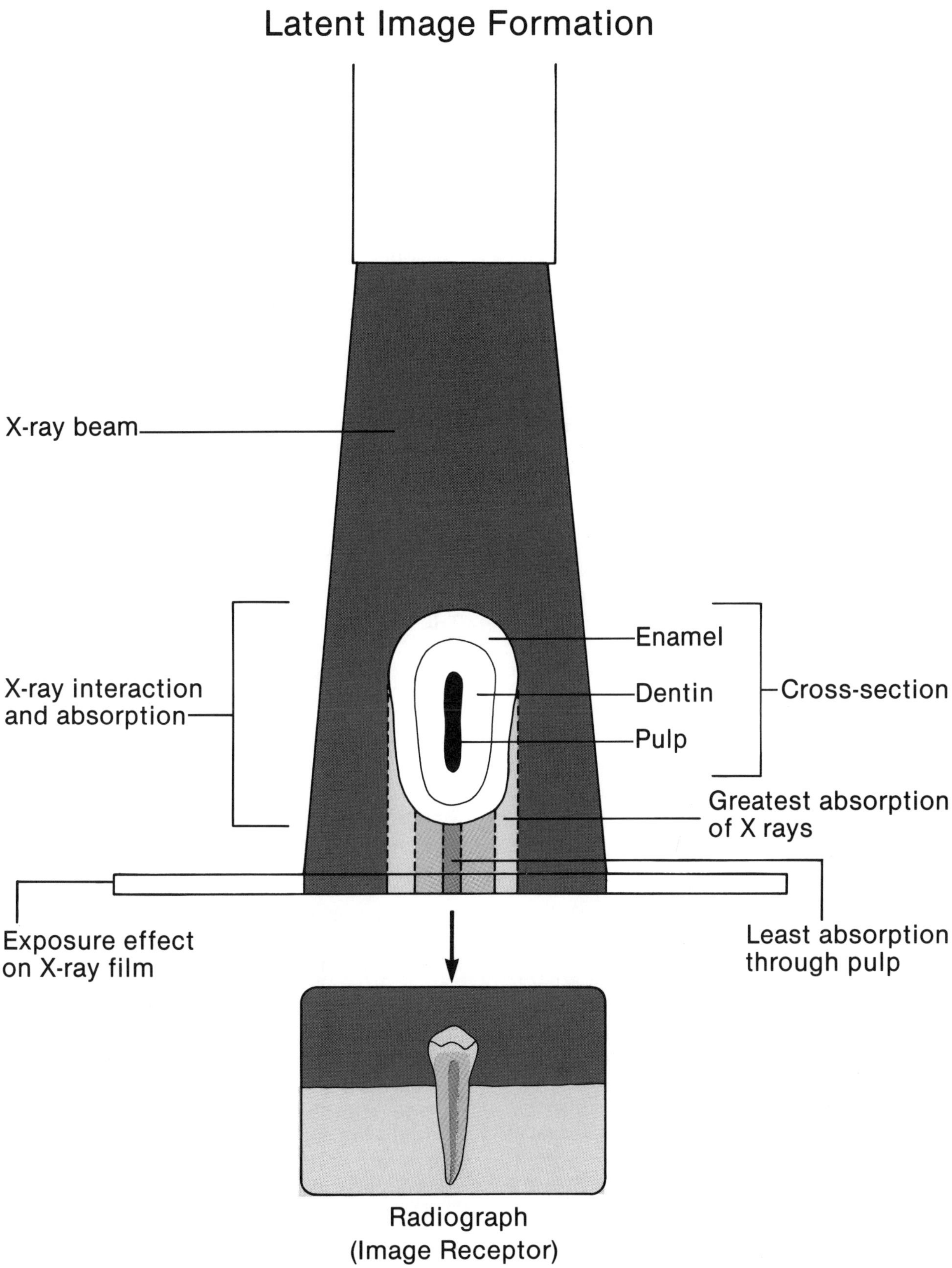

Latent Image Formation

X-ray beam

X-ray interaction and absorption

Enamel

Dentin

Pulp

Cross-section

Greatest absorption of X rays

Exposure effect on X-ray film

Least absorption through pulp

Radiograph
(Image Receptor)

Fig. 5, V-4 Latent image formation.

is to be able to recognize those characteristics related to density that impair interpretation. When too little x ray is used, there will be too little density for interpretation of the image. Where there is too much exposure, the radiograph will be too dark or dense for interpretation. The radiographer must evaluate each patient for size, then establish the amount of x rays in terms of mA, time, and kVp to expose and properly record a diagnostic image with easily distinguishable densities.

Contrast in a radiographic image is the difference between whiteness and blackness seen on the film. Final image contrast results from the combination of two factors, subject contrast and film contrast.

Subject contrast is determined by the thickness of the structures through which the x-ray beam passes, the density of the structures, and the extent that scatter radiation affects the film during exposure. Subject contrast is established on the film by the kVp setting. Because higher kVp, above 70 kVp, results in a more penetrating beam, greater variations in tissue densities are recorded in the image. These images are referred to as demonstrating low contrast because many gray shades are present between the white and black densities on the film, and only slight differences are detectible between the gray shades.

High-contrast images are produced by the use of lower kVp techniques. The high-contrast image shows only a few gray shades between the white and black areas on the film. The term "high contrast" is used because larger differences are seen in the gray steps between the white and black shadows, mainly because there are fewer gray tones present. See Figure 14, Section 1.

The dentist determines the contrast required to diagnose diseases for the patient. Once established and set on the machine, the radiographer then sets the correct mA and time settings (mAs) for that kVp. The size of the patient and the length of the cone used are also taken into consideration. See Section 1.

Film contrast is the overall contrast of the image as affected by four factors related to the film and the way it is handled: (1) the composition of the emulsion with regard to crystal size and sensitivity; (2) the density of the image recorded, resulting from the correct mAs settings; (3) whether screen or direct exposure is used; (4) the efficiency of the processing system used to develop and fix the film. Underdeveloped films or the use of exhausted or cold developer prevents normal contrast from being obtained. Overdeveloped film results in "fog," which affects visible film contrast.

Detail is often used synonymously with "definition," "sharpness," and "resolution" when referring to image quality. Although these terms actually have independent meanings, it is permissible to discuss them under the term "detail." The term refers to the capability of the film to reproduce the sharp outlines of an object. In dentistry it should be thought of as the ability of the film to distinguish small changes in tissue densities from the most radiopaque (enamel) to the most radiolucent (sinuses). Detail, as it refers to an x-ray image, is relative to the size of the crystal or grain in the emulsion. A film emulsion consisting of larger crystals has more speed or sensitivity to x-ray exposure. These have less detail because the larger crystals cannot produce object outlines as well as slower-speed film, which has smaller crystals in its emulsion. Detail will also be affected by the contrast, which depends on several key factors stated previously. Detail also depends on the implementation of the five principles of shadow casting, primarily rules 1, 2, and 3. See Section 5.

Motion of the patient during the exposure also results in the loss of detail through blurring of the image. The radiographer should instruct the patient not to move during each exposure (Fig. 6, V-4).

THE DARKROOM

Because standardizing darkroom radiographic procedures is important to image quality, a thorough discussion of the darkroom facility and policy related to its use will be given in this section.

DESIGN OF THE DARKROOM

The location of the darkroom should be convenient and within easy access of other facilities within the dental office. The room should be large enough to provide for disposal of waste materials in order to maintain cleanliness. The darkroom should have a minimum of 20 square feet of floor space to ensure that the facility is adequate for handling conventional dental x-ray processing equipment.

If the facility is utilized for storage of film, preconstruction must allow for ventilation and solid walls to protect the film emulsion from excess moisture, heat, or radiation. The room should be as cool and dry as possible. Another essential is ample storage space to accommodate film, processing chemicals, automatic processor, and tanks, as well as related materials. The room should be light-tight and easily accessible with an entrance through a rotating door, or a maze, or through a door that has an inside lock to prevent accidental exposure by other employ-

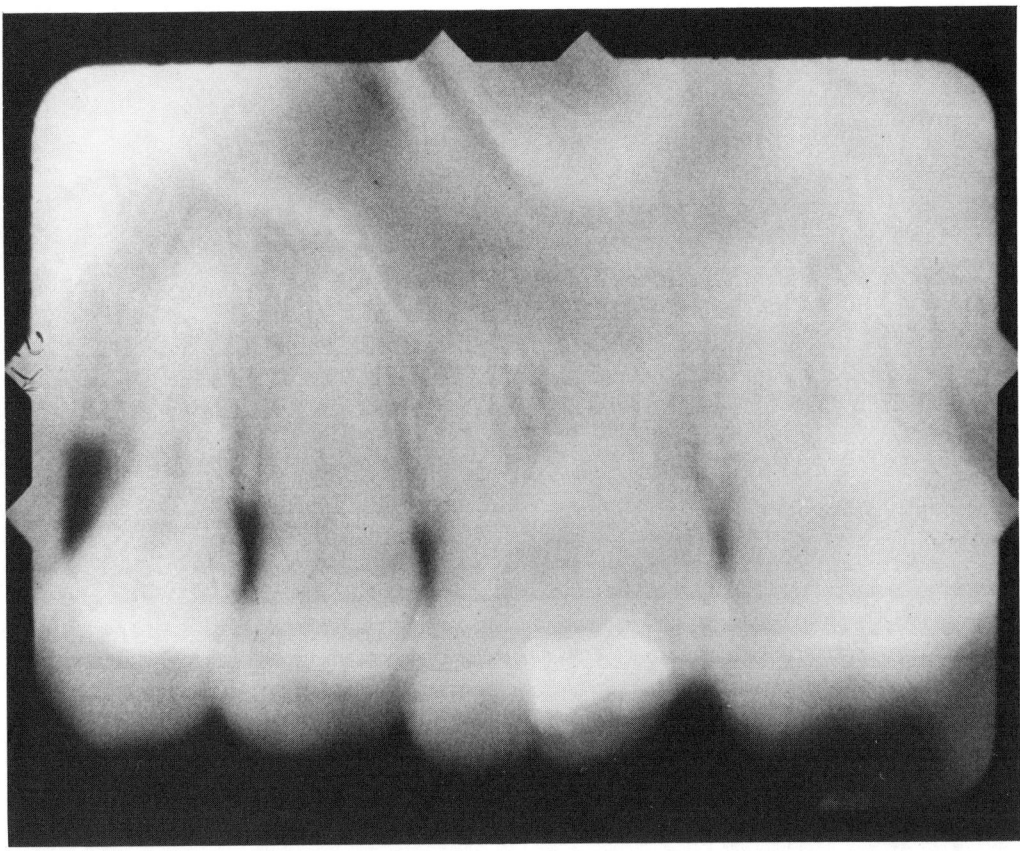

Fig. 6, V-4 Motion blurring. Results of patient, film, or tube movement.

ees during film-processing procedures. Plumbing should always include hot and cold water, needed for heating or cooling developing chemicals.

Lighting

Two types of lighting are used in the darkroom —normal and safelight. Normal room lighting is used for performing duties such as cleaning, stocking, and mixing chemicals; the safelight is used when opening and processing exposed radiographs. Accidental exposure to normal room light will "fog" the images on the film, causing them to be black. Because some visibility is needed while processing films, safelight systems are available. Normally this light is a filtered, low-wattage (approximately 15 watts) light bulb. The most appropriate safelight filter is the universal filter (GBX-2, Kodak) which allows safe handling of intraoral and extraoral film (Fig. 7A, B, V-4). Radiographers should utilize the literature available within each shipment of film, for it establishes the recommended safelight system for that particular film.

It is important to note that screen film and non-

screen film possess different sensitivity levels. If non-screen film only is used in an office, a filter that permits more light into the darkroom can be used (ML 2, Kodak). If both non-screen intraoral film and screen film such as panoramic or cephalometric radiographs are developed, the universal filter should be used. Generally the safelight should be at least 4 feet above the workbench areas where x-ray packets are opened and placed on racks or where they are placed in the feeder system of an automatic processor. Before risking damage to any image, it is wise to check the safelight and darkroom for white light leakage.

Testing the Darkroom for Light Leaks

Several tests can be used when checking for light leaks in the darkroom. After working in the darkroom for one-half hour, and when one's eyes have become completely dark-adapted, no light should be observed leaking into the room around the doors. Usually this procedure will be required only once unless the office is remodeled or reconstructed. Another test, the "penny test," is described under the Quality Assurance heading of this section.

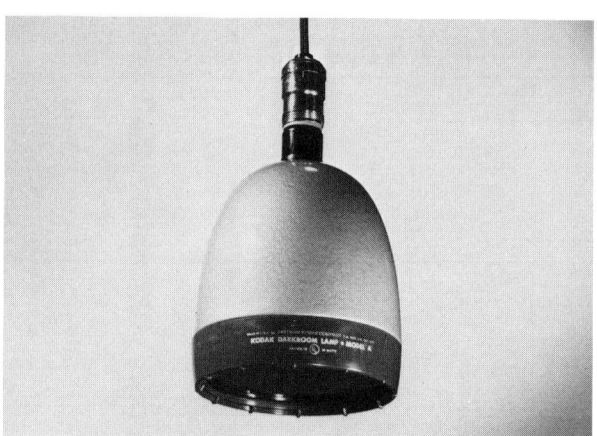

Fig. 7, V-4 Safelights.
    A. Ceiling-mounted safelight.

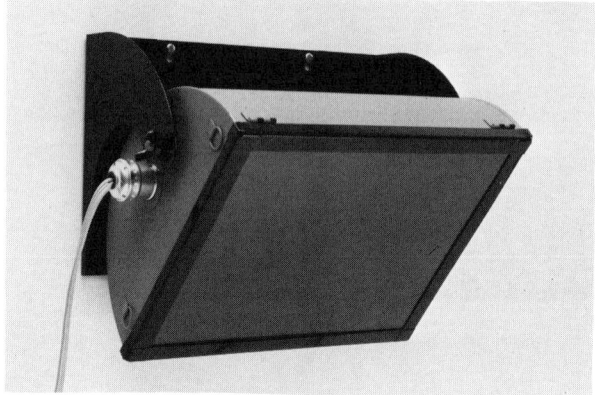

    B. Wall-mounted safelight. *(Courtesy of Eastman Kodak Co., Rochester, NY)*

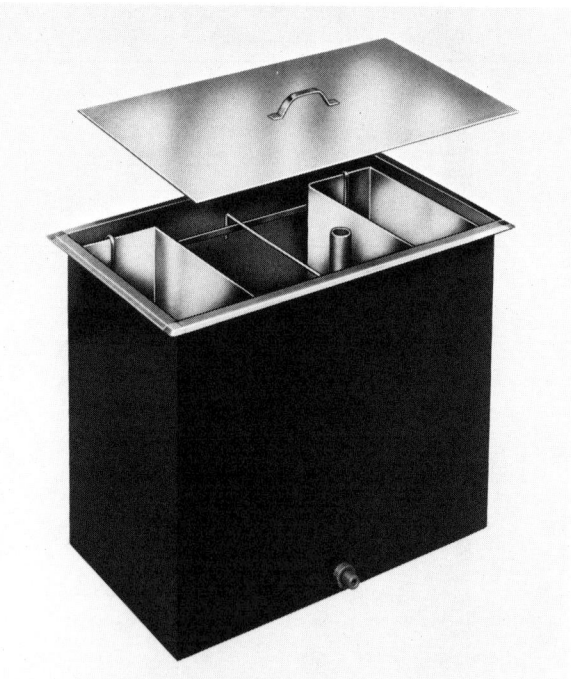

Fig. 8, V-4 Processing tanks.
    A. Five-gallon processing tank.

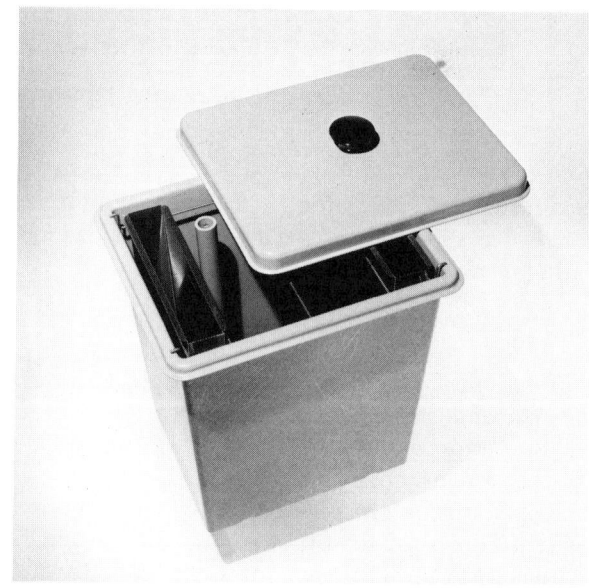

    B. One-gallon processing tank. *(Courtesy of General Electric Co., Milwaukee, WI)*

EQUIPMENT

Tanks

Many kinds of equipment are available for film processing. The developing tanks are essential items, and they are made of hard rubber, stainless steel, or plastic. It is important to label the tanks for personnel unfamiliar with the darkroom. An advantage of hard rubber tanks is that the rubber acts as an insulator to maintain the temperature of the solutions. Steel tanks are easier to clean, but they are also more expensive. Plastic, which is the least expensive of the three, is also the least desirable. Processing tanks consist of an outer tank filled with running water and two inner tanks, one each for developer and fixer solutions (Fig. 8A, B, V-4). A standpipe is installed in the water-bath section to permit excess water to pass down the drain. At the same time a higher water-

bath level is maintained between and surrounding the tank inserts for the processing solutions. Openings with stoppers are present at the bottom of the developer and fixer tanks to allow draining and cleaning when the solutions are replaced. The tank

60

lid should be kept in place except when placing or removing films in order to prevent oxidation of the processing chemicals.

The maintenance of the temperature of the developer is a very important factor in processing films correctly. The temperature of the solutions is controlled by the temperature of the circulating water. Reliable maintenance of the water temperature is achieved by means of a mixing valve, which functions in a way similar to those found in bathroom showers. The incoming hot and cold water are mixed so that the water flowing through the bath is 68°F.

Accessories

For tasks such as mixing chemicals and cleaning, a large sink is needed. It is recommended that it be a porcelain, flush-mounted sink or a stainless steel sink with a mixing faucet. In some cases a hose can be attached to the faucet for the purpose of running water around the developer tank to maintain the 68°F solution temperatures. This is important for temperature regulation when refrigeration units are not available.

An adequate number of stainless steel hangers should be available above the workbench. The hangers come in many sizes, varying from one film clip to a dozen or more, and should be no longer than the depth of the developing tanks (Fig. 9, V-4).

For constant monitoring of the temperatures of the chemical solutions thermometers of special design are available. The recommended thermometers are made of stainless steel or glass. Regular thermometers are not suitable for this purpose because of the corrosive action of the chemicals in which they remain immersed.

Stirring rods, paddles, and funnels of glass and plastic are utilized for daily stirring of solutions. Other materials are not suitable for this use because of the corrosive action of the processing chemicals. Plastic aprons should be available in the darkroom to protect clothing during processing and mixing of chemicals. A clock with a loud alarm for time-temperature processing should also be included (Fig. 10, V-4).

Care of the Equipment

Cleanliness is essential. Mineral salts and carbonate deposits that form on the walls of processing tanks may be removed by soaking the containers with a cold or lukewarm solution of 1.5 ounces of hydrochloric (muriatic) acid to 1 gallon of water for a 1-gallon tank. The procedure may be repeated as often as mixing in the tank is desired. Rinsing

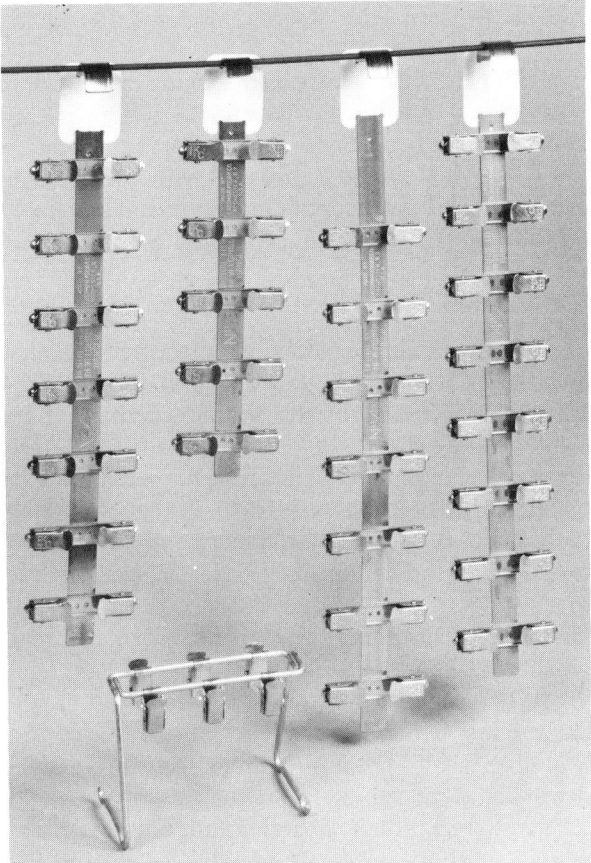

Fig. 9, V-4 Processing racks.

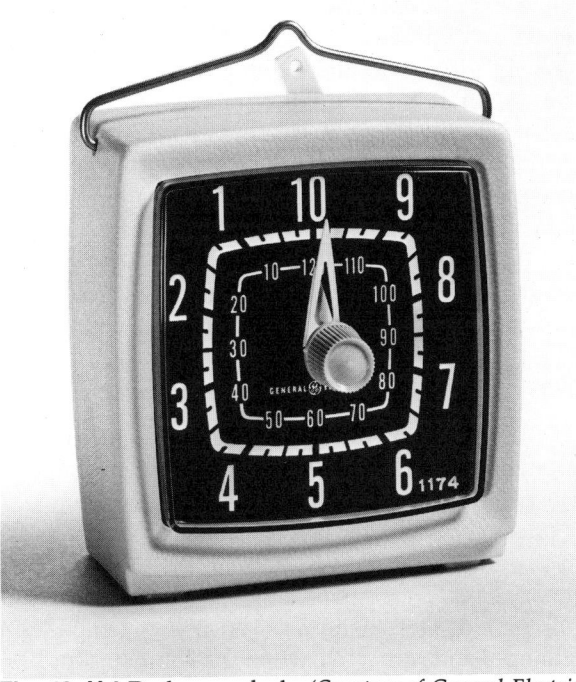

Fig. 10, V-4 Darkroom clock. (*Courtesy of General Electric Co., Milwaukee, WI*)

thoroughly with fresh water is essential after each soaking.

Hangers can be cleaned by soaking in a solution of 1/8 ounce of trypsin, 1/8 ounce of sodium bicarbonate, and 1 gallon of water for 1/2 hour at 100–125°F. They should be brushed with a wire brush (especially if they are corroded), resoaked in a fresh solution, and then washed thoroughly.

Storage and Preparation of Darkroom Solutions

It is important to follow manufacturers' recommendations when storing, mixing, and utilizing radiographic solutions. In the average dental office, solutions are usually exhausted approximately every two weeks, and in an office with a higher volume of patients it may be necessary to change solutions more often. Solutions should be covered to prevent oxidation of the chemicals. Oxidation is a process that results in a breakdown of the chemicals in solution, thus shortening the length of time during which they can be used.

When preparing solutions it is important to follow the instructions available in printed form or on container labels. These solutions can be ordered in dry or liquid concentrates. Particular attention should be paid to recommended water temperatures when mixing solutions. Separate paddles for stirring the developer and fixer are utilized and should be clearly identified by color or label to prevent leftover fixer from contaminating new developer. The resulting error is exhausted developer, which must be disposed of immediately. Unused chemicals (those not yet mixed) should be stored in a cool, dry location. Extra solutions for replenishment may be stored in the same manner and utilized daily to maintain the working strength and tank levels of the solutions. Special replenishments of solutions can also be purchased for this purpose.

Each chemical in the developer and fixer has an important role in producing an optimum final product.

Developer

The developer is made up of the following components:

1. Reducing agents:

a. *Hydroquinone* is a reducer that blackens the exposed silver halide crystals. It acts slowly but the image gains density steadily throughout the developing period. This chemical is sensitive to temperature changes and is inactive when the solution drops below 60°F. It is primarily responsible for bringing out the contrast.

b. *Elon* is a reducer that blackens exposed crystals. It is made from a by-product of dyes treated with methyl alcohol. Elon gives detail to the image. It is not affected by slight temperature changes.

2. Alkalizer: *Sodium carbonate* is the component that provides the required alkaline medium in which the reducers work. It swells and softens the gelatin in the emulsion, allowing the reducing agents to reach the silver bromide crystals.

3. Preservative: *Sodium sulfite* is the preservative agent that slows the oxidation and subsequent spoilage of the developing solution. This increases the life span of the solution to two to four weeks.

4. Restrainer: *Potassium bromide* slows down the action of chemicals in solution to a practical speed, thereby preventing chemical fog.

5. *Distilled water* is the vehicle used to mix these chemicals.

Fixer

The fixer not only stops the actions of the developing solutions but also removes unexposed and undeveloped crystals that are unaffected by the developer.

The chemicals in the fixer are as follows:

1. *Sodium* or *ammonium thiosulfate* or *hyposulfate* is known as the "hypo" agent and is the chemical that removes the unexposed and/or undeveloped crystals from the film.

2. *Acetic acid* provides the required acidity so that fixing solutions can work. It also stops the developing action.

3. *Sodium sulfite* works in the same manner as in the developer.

4. *Potassium alum* shrinks and hardens the emulsion. It also protects the emulsion from abrasion and aids rapid drying of the film.

5. *Distilled water* is the vehicle for mixing these solutions.

QUALITY ASSURANCE

Quality assurance refers to "the routine and special procedures developed to ensure that the final radiographic product is of a consistently high quality." The radiographer plays an important role in this process and is encouraged to periodically review the technical quality of the radiographs with other staff members. A second responsibility of the radiographer involves making arrangements for periodic equipment inspection by state and local regulatory agencies. Items assessed during this process include

(1) timer and milliamperage accuracy, (2) the x-ray tube for possible leakage of radiation, and (3) the collimation and alignment of the x-ray beam.

Quality assurance of procedures that relate to film processing include a periodic evaluation of the darkroom for light leaks and implementation of the "penny test" (Table 1, V-4) to document correct safelight illumination. Routine equipment checks and monitoring procedures include (1) weekly cleaning of automatic roller assembly and manual-system film racks, (2) records of daily and weekly maintenance procedures, (3) daily monitoring of solution temperatures and levels, and (4) sensitometric analysis for fog, speed, and contrast.

Table 1, V-4

1. Place a coin on an unwrapped, unexposed piece of x-ray film.
2. Place coin and film on work counter below safelight for 2 to 3 minutes.
3. Process film using standard procedure.
4. View film for outline of the coin.
5. If coin image is visible on film, safelight is inadequate.

A simple system that aids the radiographer in establishing an effective quality-assurance program is the "Dental Radiographic Normalizing and Monitoring Device" (Fig. 11A, B, V-4). This system can be used to "reduce the number of retakes, track skin x-ray dose per film, minimize duplication in radiographic services, signal a need to change solutions, and detect deficiencies before film quality is degraded." More information about the system is available from Dental Radiographic Devices.

PATIENT IDENTIFICATION

Correct identification of a patient's film is obviously very important. If intraoral films are processed manually, the rack used should be labeled with the patient's name in one of several possible ways: (1) the lead foil inside a film packet can be labeled and then wrapped around the stem of the rack used for that patient's films; (2) the actual plastic film packet can be used in the same manner and clipped to the rack; or (3) there are commercially available plastic labels that slide onto the rack.

If intraoral films are automatically processed, a system of envelopes labeled with the patient's name can be used to avoid confusion. The films can be stored in the envelopes until processing, and then, as the radiographs are placed in the automatic processor, the labeled envelopes can be placed in order corresponding to the film's exit from the processor. A blank film can be processed between the different sets of films to help identify each patient's radiographs.

Whichever method of processing or labeling is used, it is of the utmost importance that the patient's identification remain intact through the point of mounting and labeling with name and date.

When extraoral films are taken, the name and date are "flashed" on the film using a device called a film flasher (Fig. 12, V-4). The information is writ-

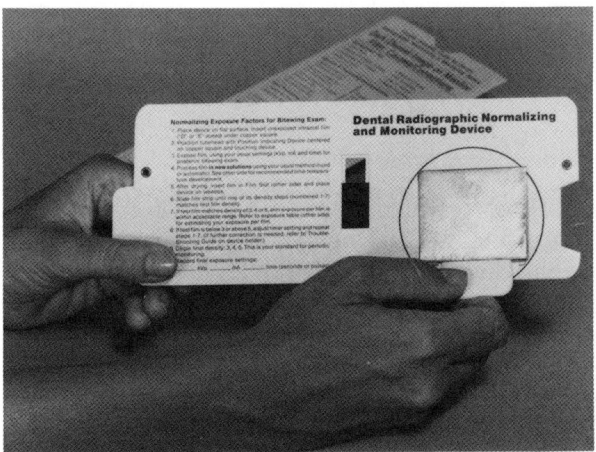
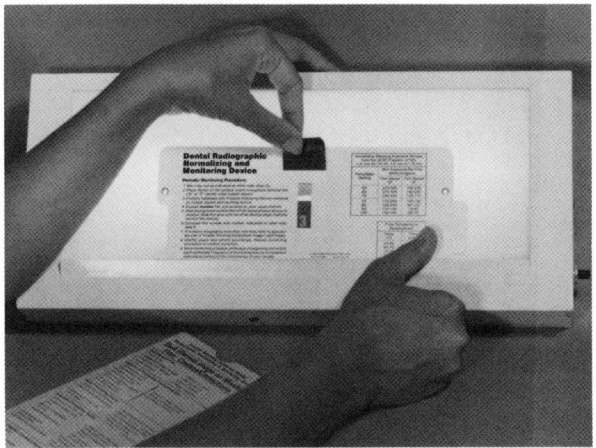

Fig. 11, V-4 Dental radiographic normalizing and monitoring device.
A. Preparing to expose film packet.

B. Comparing quality of processed film. (*Courtesy of Dental Radiographic Devices, Silver Spring, MD*)

Fig. 12, V-4 Patient identification.

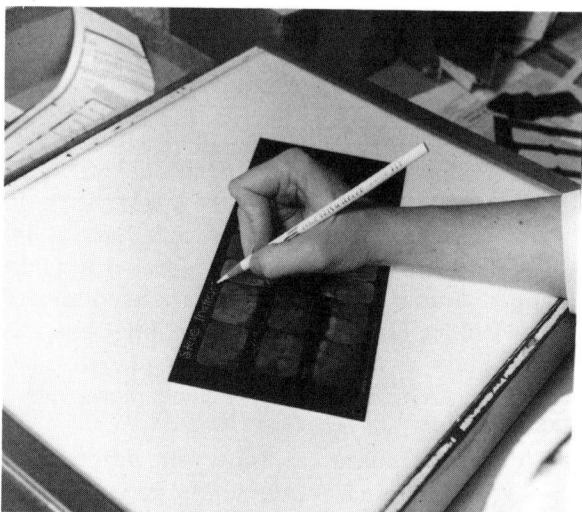

A. Patient's name and the date are written on the mount for intraoral films.

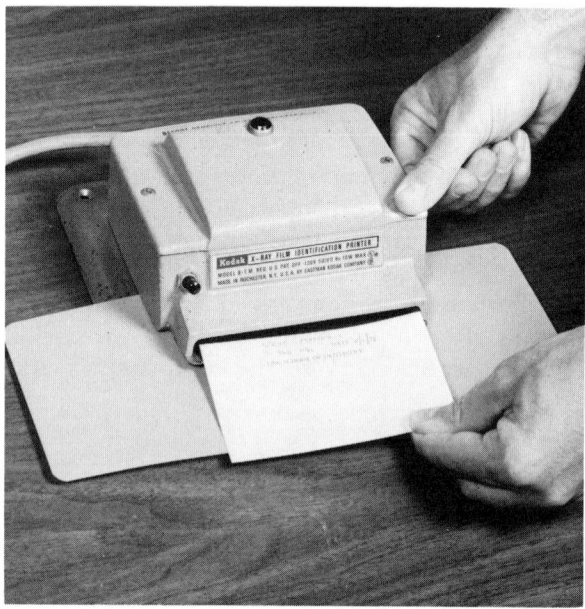

B. Film flasher used for extraoral film.

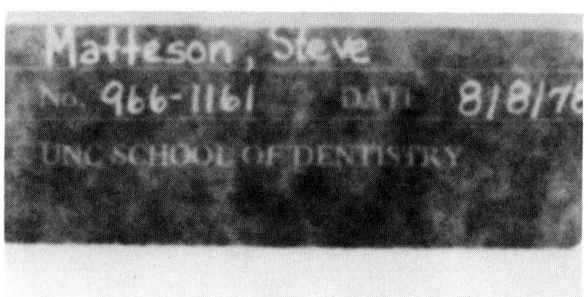

C. Patient information becomes part of film image.

ten on a card and after the film is exposed, the film and card are placed in the flasher. The exposure bar is pressed to activate a small light which shines through the card, registering the information on the film. After processing, the name and date can be seen in the film image. This method is generally better than writing the name and date on the film with a pen, as the latter may be accidentally removed. If lead letters are available, they may be attached to the front of the cassette before exposure in order to imprint the name and date on the film.

PROCESSING METHODS

Automatic Processors

Automatic processors are used in many dental offices today. These are available in many styles from various manufacturers (Fig. 13A, B, V-4). This equipment has several advantages:

1. Use of the processor is convenient because films are fed directly into the machine, thus avoiding the use of racks and developing tanks.

2. Use of the processor saves time because the films are completely processed and dried in about 5 minutes compared to about 1 hour for conventional wet-tank methods.

The processors consist of sets of rollers that transport the film through the developer, fixer, and wash tanks, and then through a dryer area (Fig. 14, V-4). The process cycle is faster than the standard tank system because the temperature of the developer and fixer is held at 80°F, which accelerates the process. Special solutions are used in the automatic processors with the designation R.P. (rapid processing) (Fig. 15A, B, V-4).

Automatic processors require careful, regular maintenance, including cleaning the rollers according to the manufacturer's instructions.

Manual Processing

The recommended method of wet-tank film processing is called the *time-temperature method*. The period during which film is placed in the developer solution is timed, with the specific time period established according to the temperature of the solution. Optimum developing occurs when the temperature of the solution is 68°F. Table 2, V-4 lists the recommended times for various solutions. Temperatures lower than 60°F are too cool for film development due to inactivation of the hydroquinone. Standard dental x-ray developer and fixer are used in the wet-tank processing systems (Fig. 16, V-4).

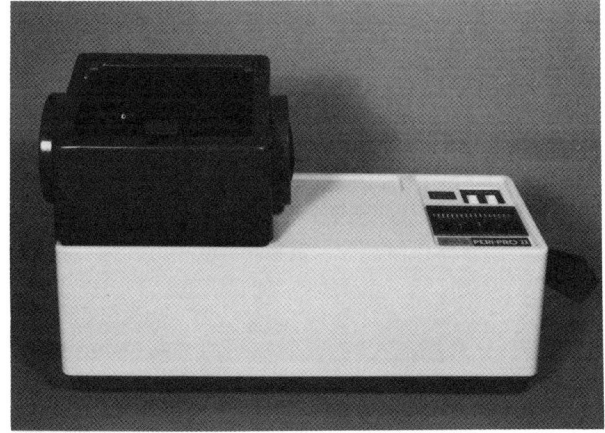

Fig. 13, V-4 Automatic processors.
A. Periapical automatic processor.

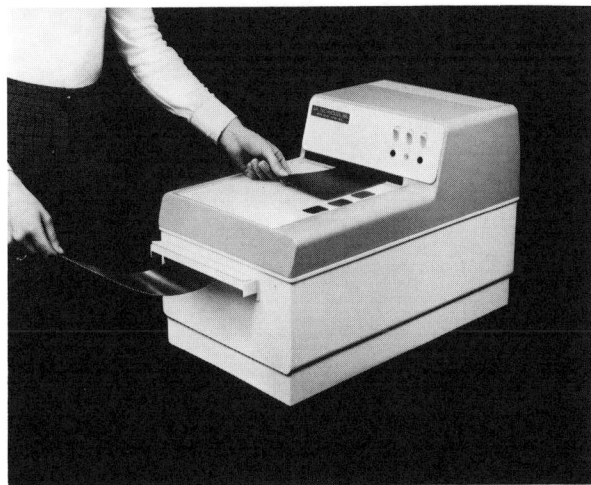

B. Processor for all sizes of films, periapical through 8-in. × 10-in. sizes. *(Courtesy of Air Technique, Inc., Hicksville, NY)*

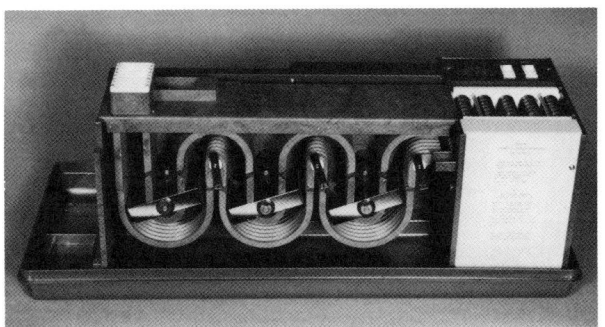

Fig. 14, V-4 Internal mechanism of an automatic processor. *(Courtesy of Air Technique, Inc., Hicksville, NY)*

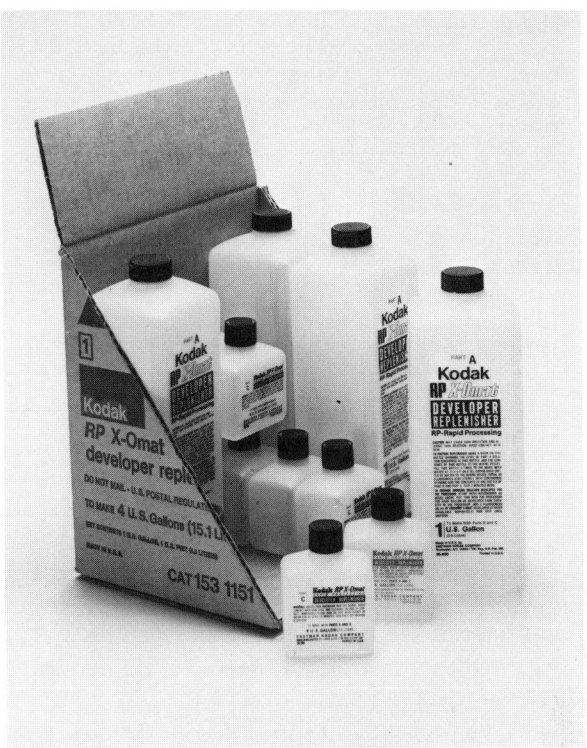

Fig. 15, V-4 Chemicals for automatic processors.
A. Developer.

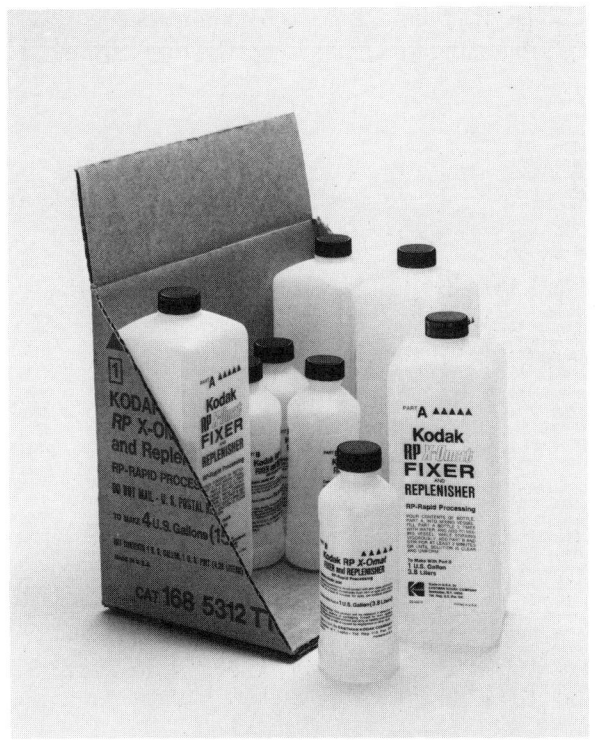

B. Fixer. *(Courtesy of Eastman Kodak Co., Rochester, NY)*

Table 2, V-4

Temperature of Developer (°F)	Time in Developer (min)
60	8
65	5½
68	4½ optimum
70	4
75	3
80	2¼

To prepare the film for processing, unwrap it and attach it by the corner with the embossed dot to the clip on a rack. Always avoid touching the surface of the film with the fingers by handling the film by its edges. Immerse the film in the developer with an agitating motion. This motion eliminates air bubbles that can keep developer from reaching the film and resulting in a film artifact. At the end of the preset developing time, remove the film rack from the developing solution and rinse in running water for 30 seconds. The rinsing action prevents contamination of the fixer bath with developer solution. Immerse the film in the fixer bath for 10 minutes, wash for 20 minutes in running water, and dry in a dust-free area over a pan or in a dryer.

Use of a timing device is recommended to measure processing times precisely. The timer shown in

Figure 17, V-4 is equipped with a preset mechanism for setting the needed time with the darkroom lights on before the films are placed on the racks. When the racks are placed in the developer or fixer, the starter level is cocked and the timer begins to run. A bell signifies the end of the preset time. Processing procedures are shown in Figure 18A–P, V-4.

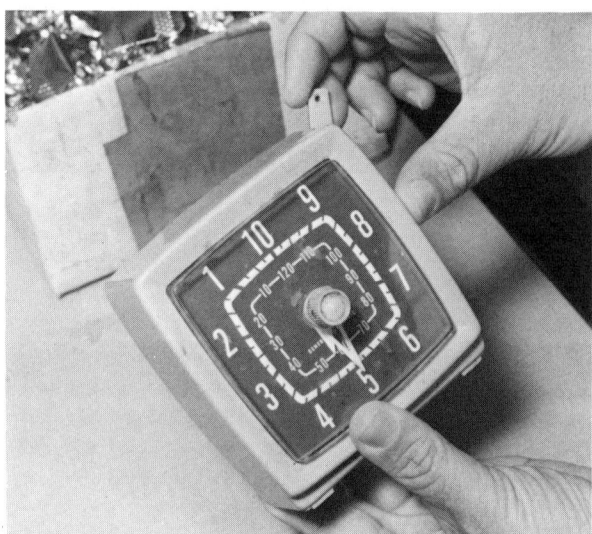

Fig. 17, V-4 Timer. *(Courtesy of Eastman Kodak Co., Rochester, NY)*

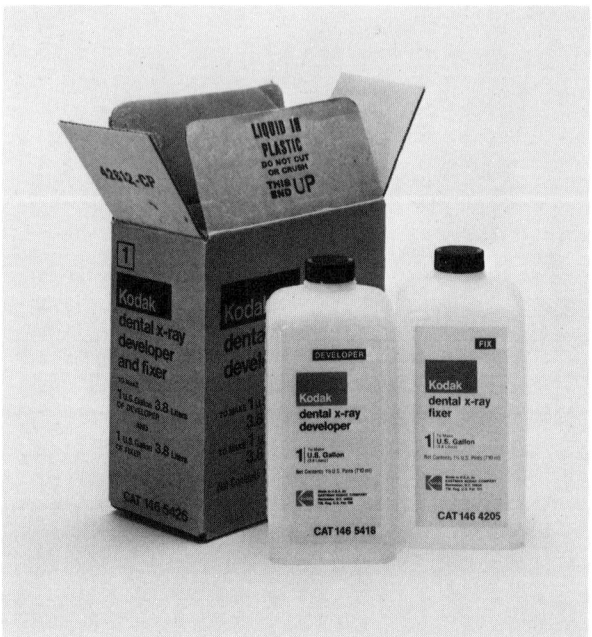

Fig. 16, V-4 Wet tank developer and fixer. *(Courtesy of Eastman Kodak Co., Rochester, NY)*

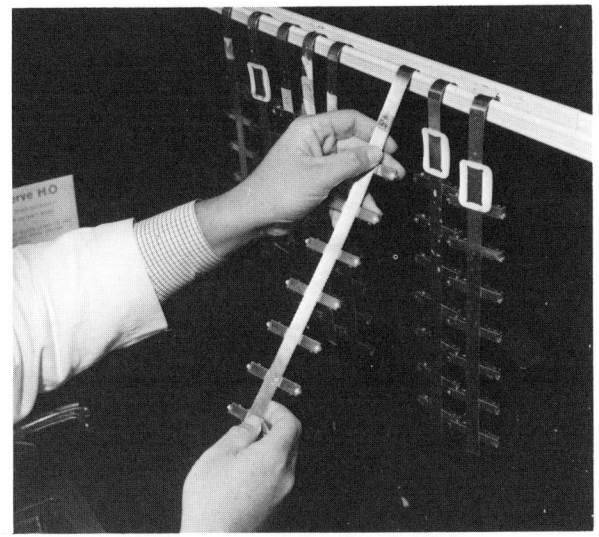

Fig. 18, V-4 Wet-tank processing procedures.
   A. Select rack for processing.

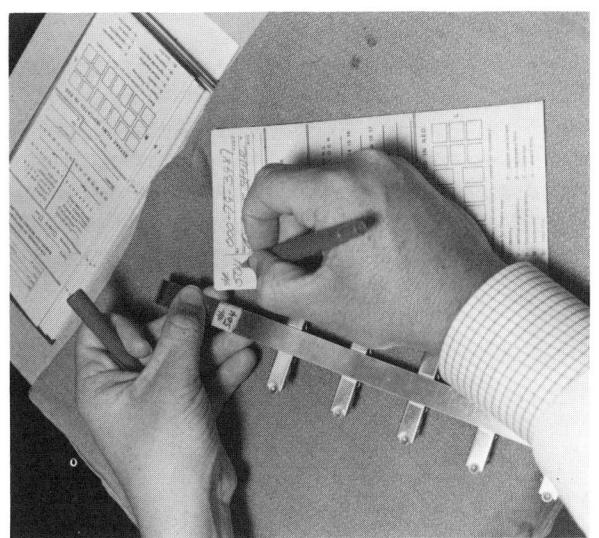

B. Record rack number on patient envelope.

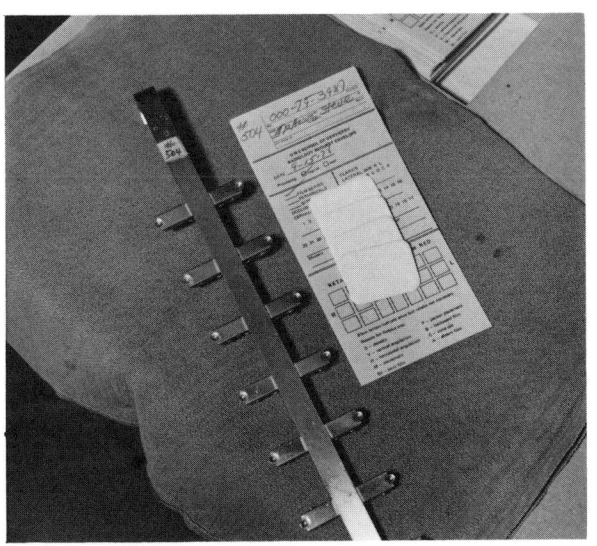

C. Assemble materials prior to entering darkroom.

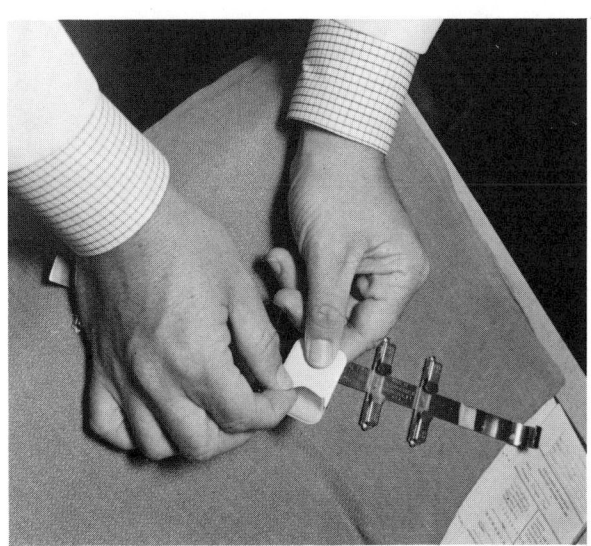

D. Open packet by pulling tab.

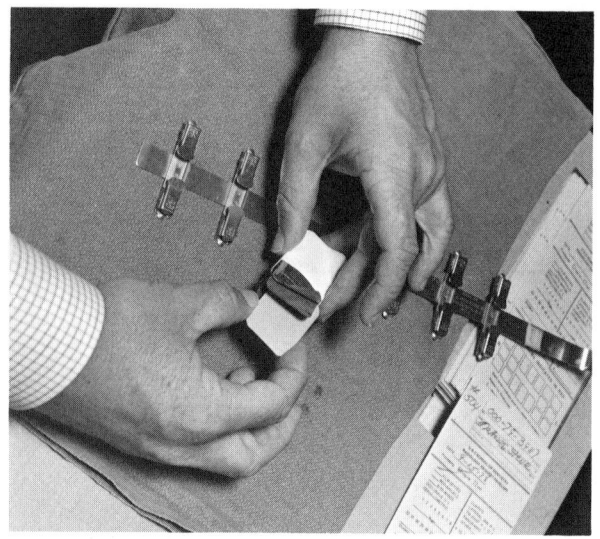

E. Separate film from contents of packet.

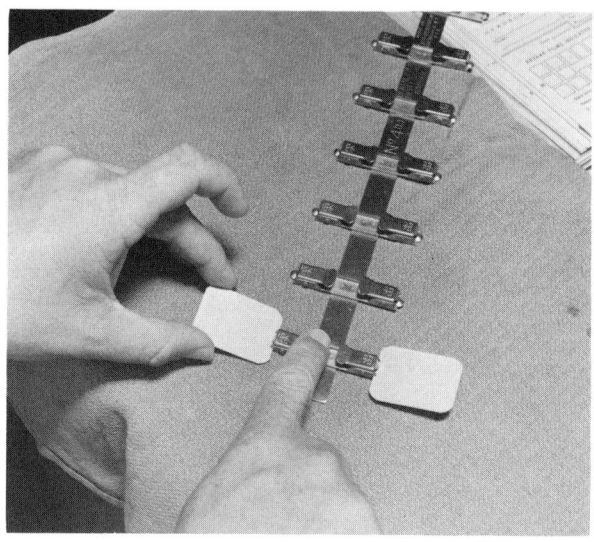

F. Attach film to metal clips.

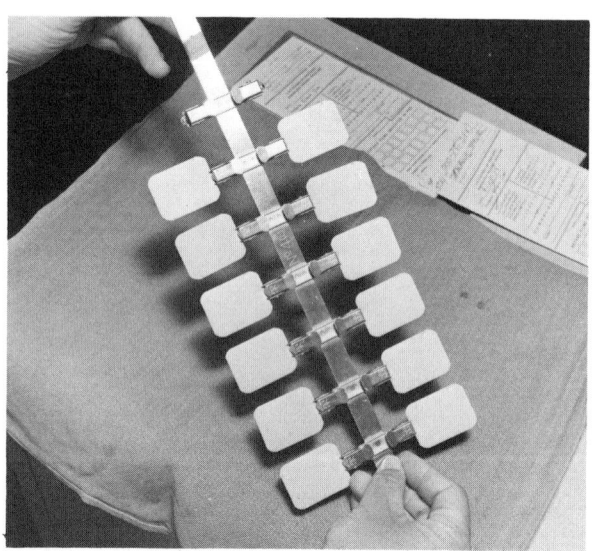

G. Rack with films in place. To avoid partial development resulting from low solution levels, top clips should not be used.

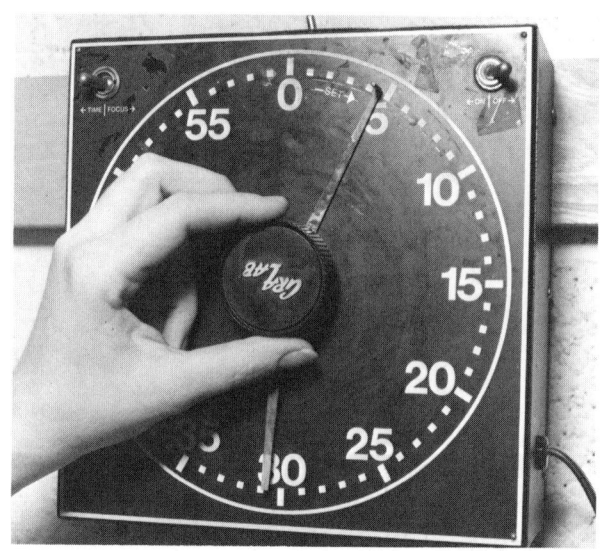

H. Set clock for 4½ minutes.

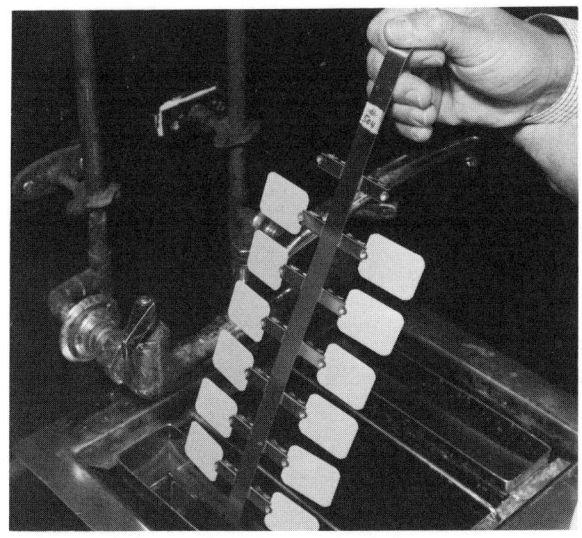

I. Immerse films in developer.

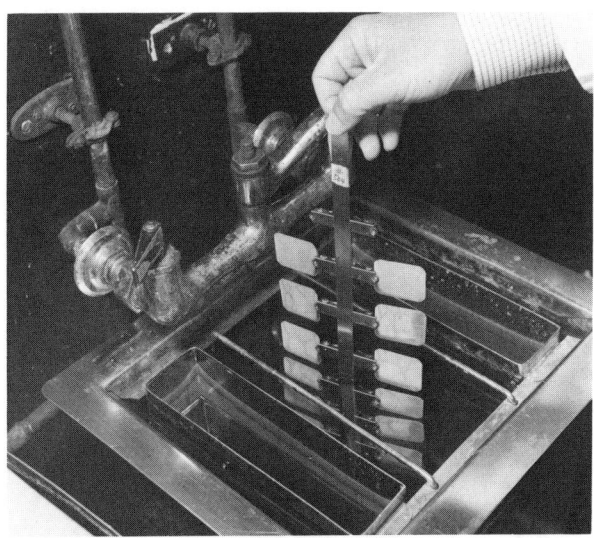

J. Rinse films for 30 seconds following developing.

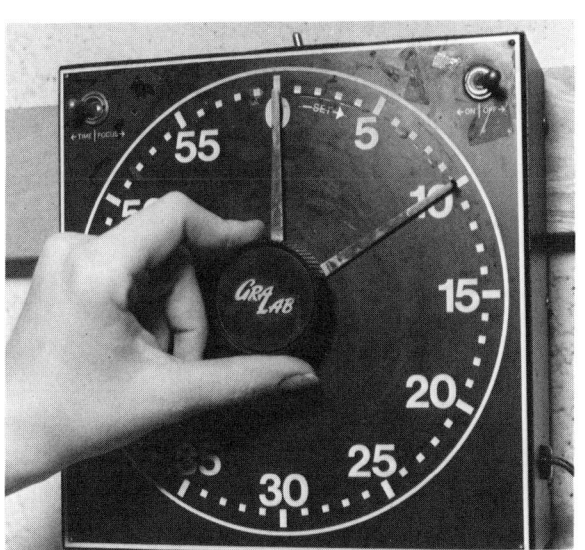

K. Set fixing times for 10 minutes.

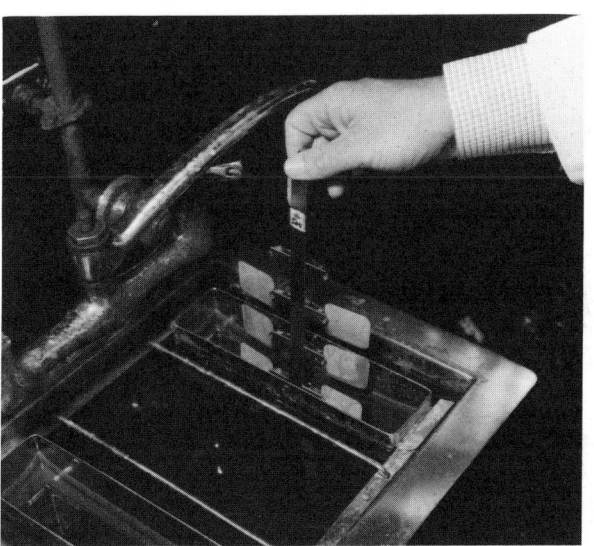

L. Immerse films in fixer.

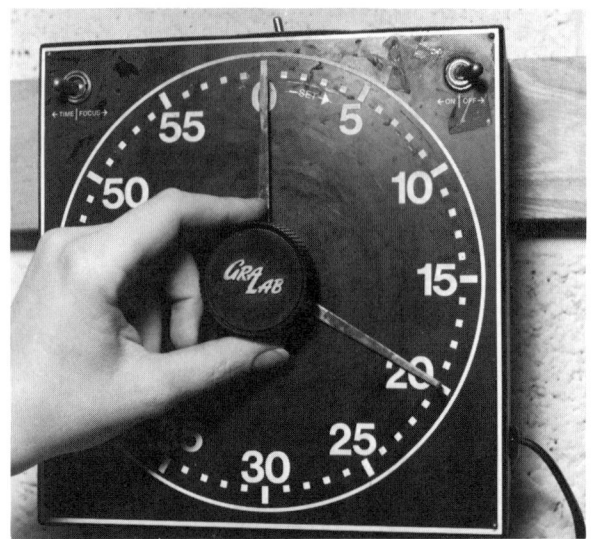

M. Set clock for 20 minutes.

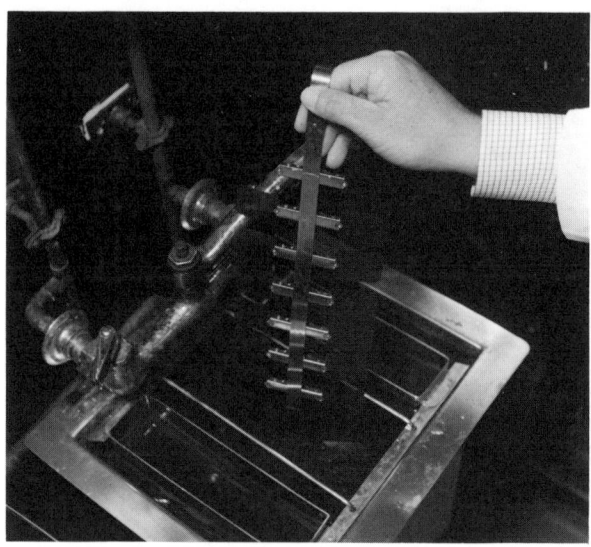

N. Immerse films in wash.

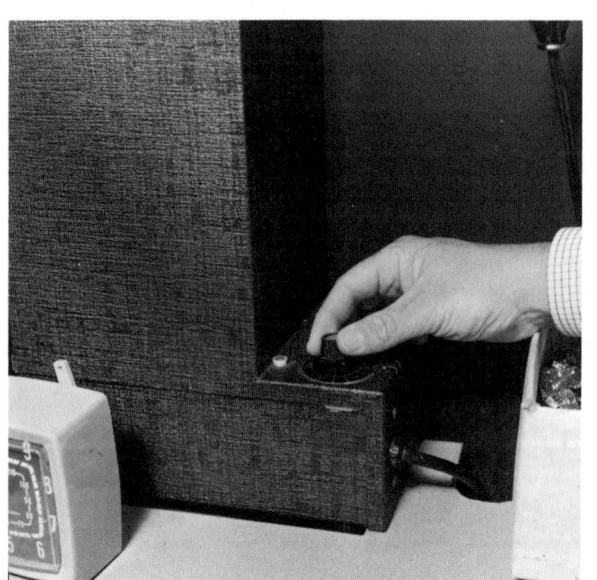

O. Set drying time for 30 minutes.

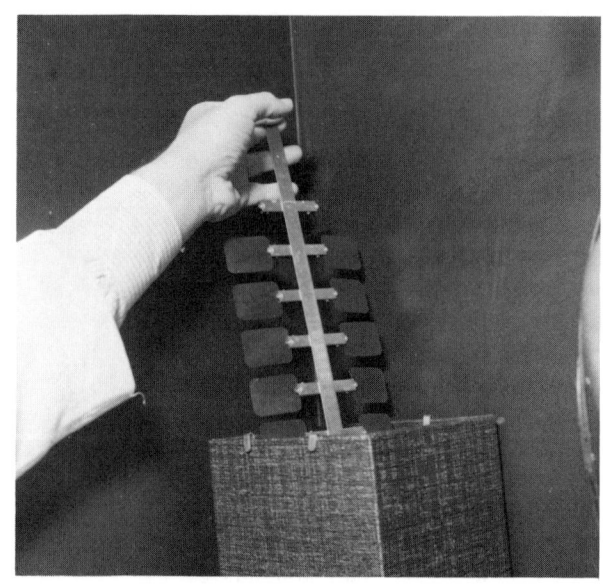

P. Place films in dryer.

PROCESSING PITFALLS

In Figures 19–22, V-4 films with processing errors are shown. Recognition of common errors is helpful in determining and correcting their cause.

Fig. 19, V-4 Results of correct and incorrect time-temperature processing.

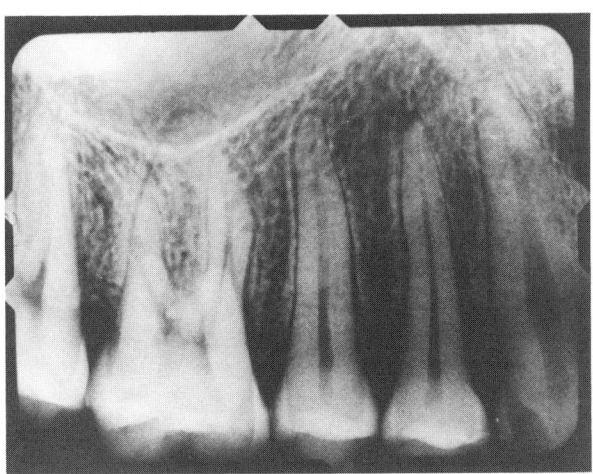

A. Correctly developed.

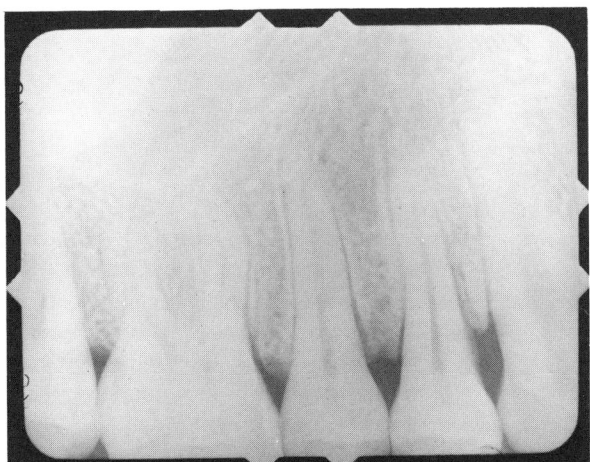

B. Underdeveloped; Possible causes:
   1. Developer temperature too low.
   2. Developing time too short.
   3. Old chemicals.

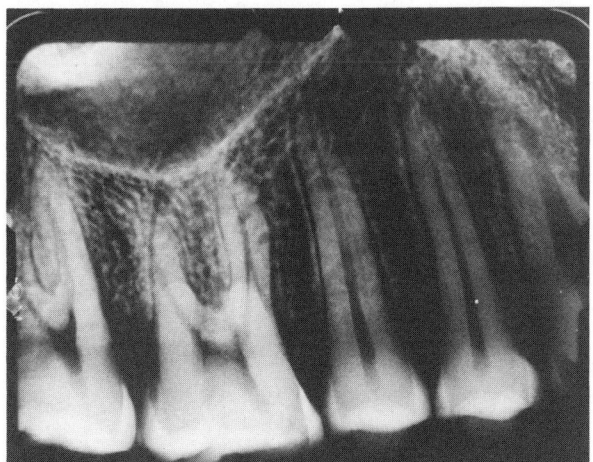

C. Overdeveloped; Possible causes:
   1. Developer temperature too high.
   2. Developing time too long.
   3. Incorrectly mixed chemicals.

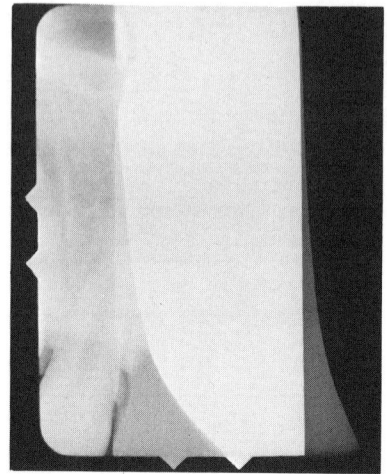

Fig. 20, V-4 Pitfalls in processing.

A. Developer level too low.

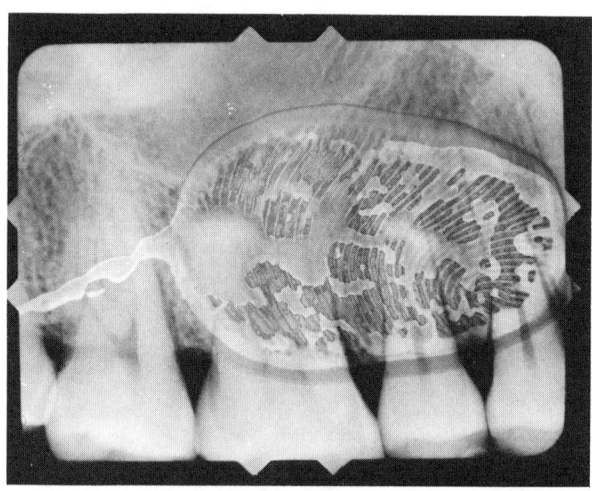

Fig. 21, V-4 Fixing pitfalls.

A. Fixer solution from thumb dissolved emulsion before development, leaving thumbprint.

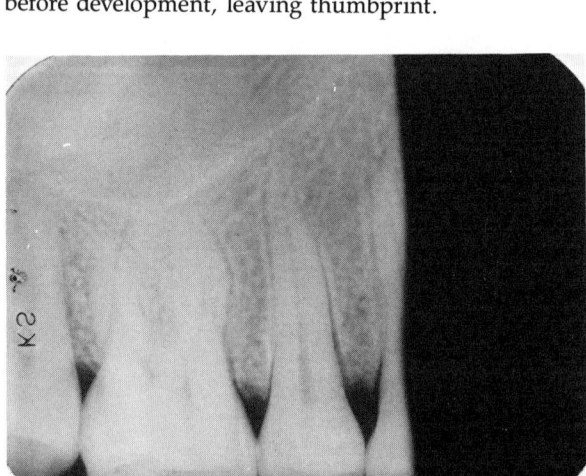

Fig. 22, V-4 Room light fog.

A. Radiograph partially "fogged" from opening.

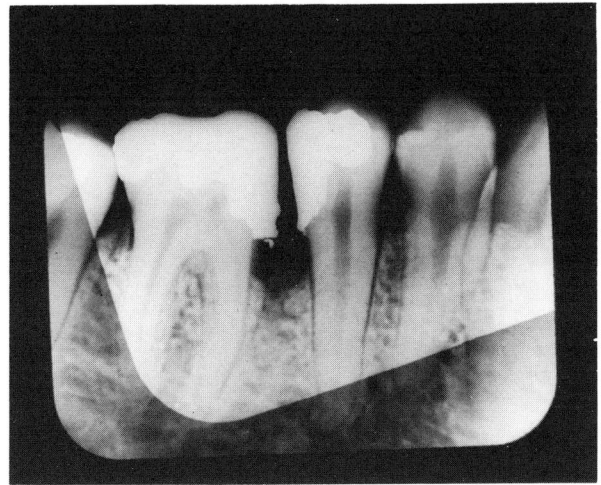

B. Films of adjacent racks overlapped during development.

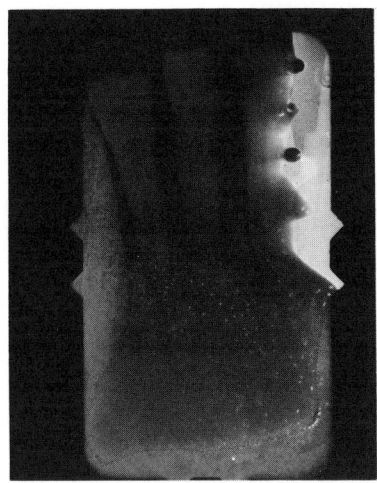

C. Original and duplicate films not separated before development.

B. Film accidentally placed in fixer prior to developing removed emulsion, leaving only film base.

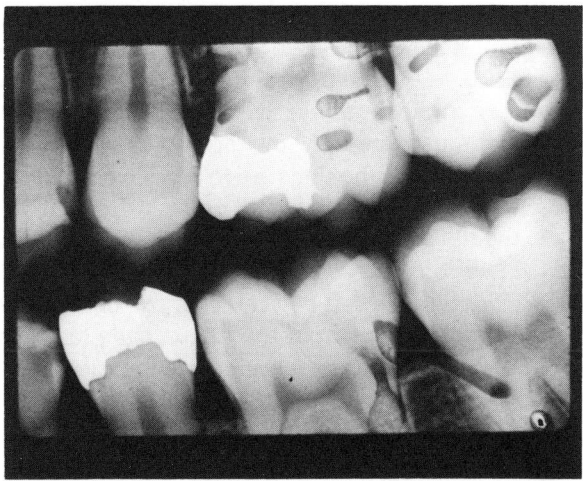

C. Insufficiently fixed and/or washed films stain with time.

B. Result of totally unwrapping film in room light, then processing.

RECORD KEEPING

Correct patient identification and filing of radiographs are important procedures which ensure that the films of each patient can be retrieved when needed. Envelopes are used to store the exposed film packets before processing and then after the films are developed. If double film packets are used, an additional envelope is required for storage of the duplicate set of films. Film duplicates are useful when patients are referred to specialists or for sending a set of radiographs to insurance companies (Fig. 23, V-4).

FILM MOUNTING

Films are routinely placed in mounts for viewing. Mounts are available with a variety of arrangements of the films. Some provide slots for holding each film, whereas other styles provide gummed paper to hold the radiographs. Because the films may be placed in the mount in two ways, the dental radiographer must determine the method used in the individual office. If the films are to be viewed as if the observer is seeing the patient from in front of the face, the films are placed in the mount with the convex side of the embossed dot up (toward the viewer). If the films are to be seen as if the observer is viewing the patient from the lingual side (as seen from the tongue), the films are placed in the mount with the concave side of the dot up (Fig. 24, V-4).

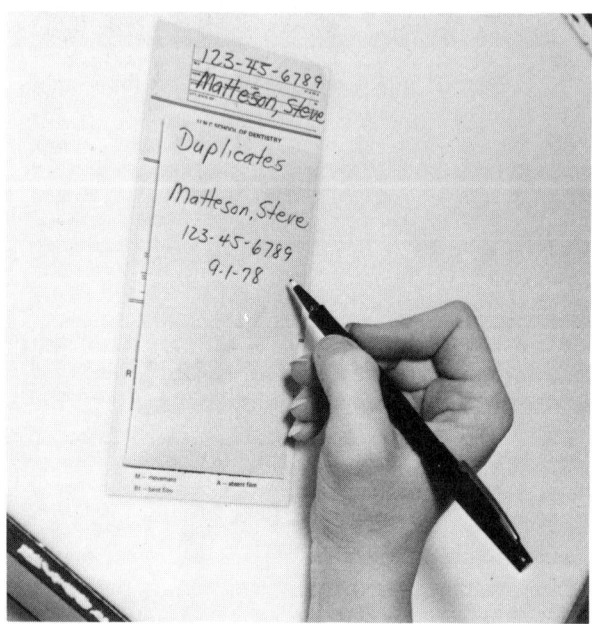

Fig. 23, V-4 Duplicate radiographs must be labeled and filed for future reference.

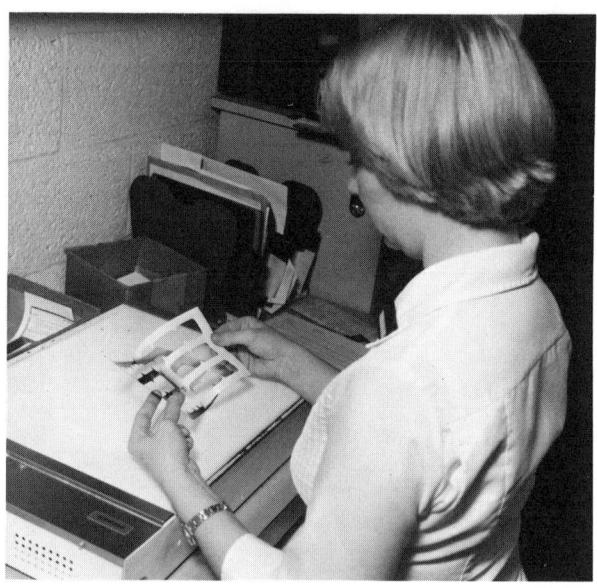

Fig. 24, V-4 Film mounting.
A. Various types of mounts are available, designed to meet individual office needs.

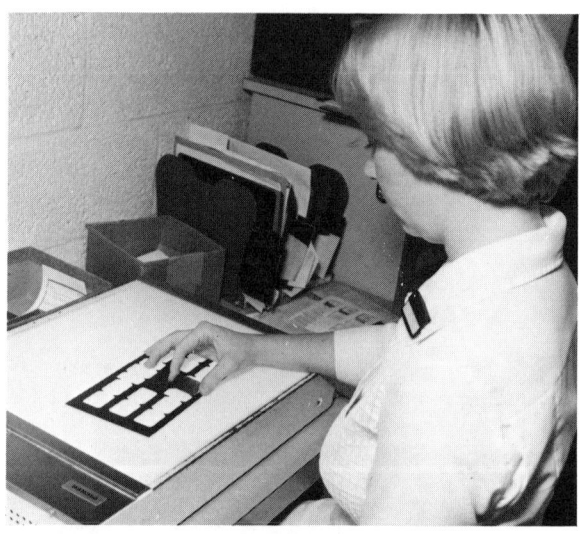

B. When mounting, use the system consistent with the office in which employed.

FILM VIEWING

Radiographs are placed on a viewbox for proper viewing (Fig. 25, V-4). Several factors are important for ideal viewing: (1) the view box should have bright, even lighting; (2) the film mounts should mask extraneous light; (3) the viewbox should be masked to prevent light other than that viewed through the radiographs from reaching the viewers'

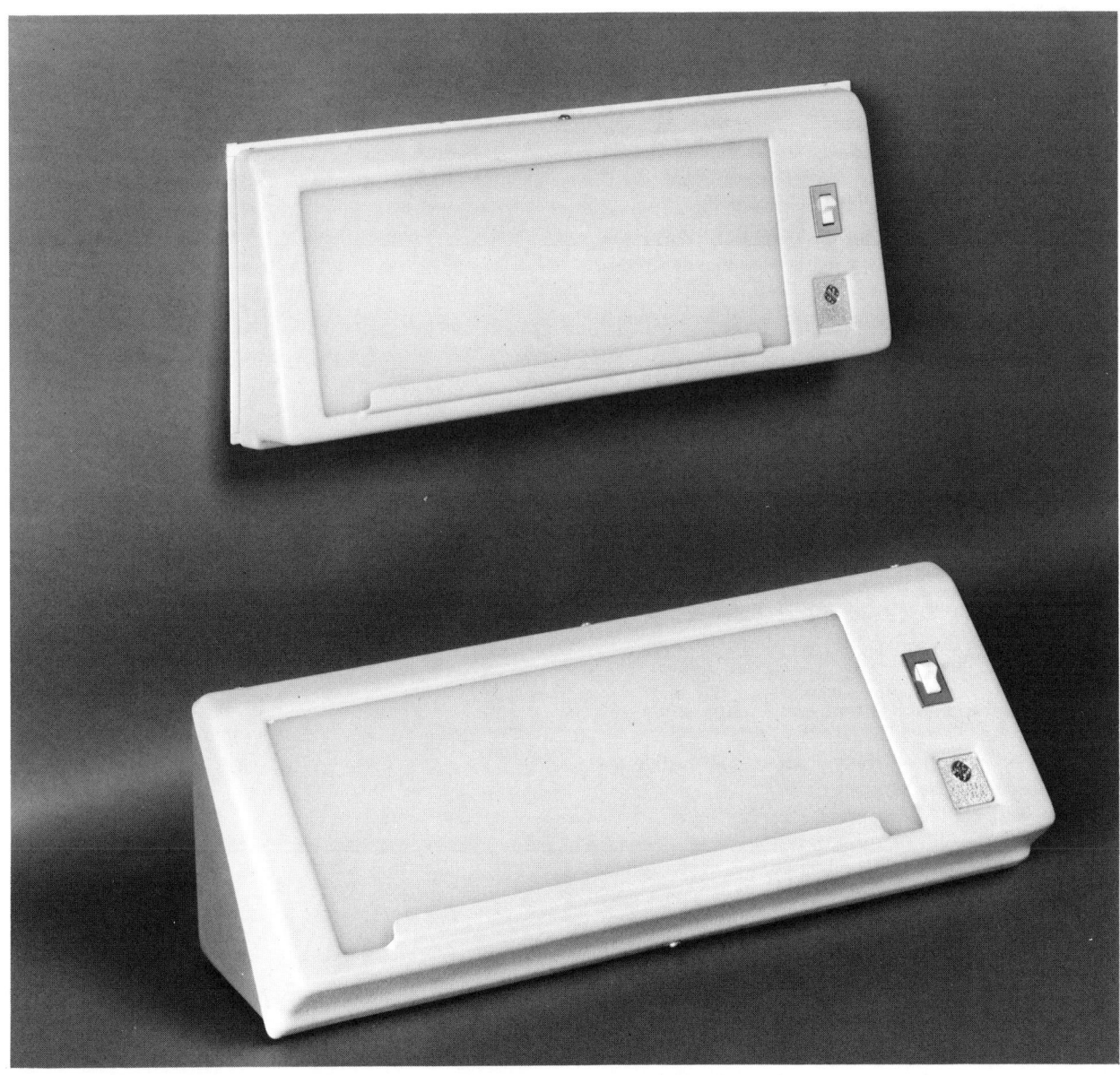

Fig. 25, V-4 Viewboxes. Top: Wall-mounted. Bottom: Desk-style.

eyes; and (4) the room lights where films are viewed should be dimmed. These simple viewing practices can be arranged by the dental radiographer to provide maximum diagnostic information from each radiograph interpreted by the dentist.

BIBLIOGRAPHY

Curry, T. S., III; Dowdey, J. E.; and Murry, R. C., Jr. *Christensen's Physics of Diagnostic Radiology*. 4th ed. Philadelphia: Lea & Febiger, 1990.

De Lyre, W. R., and Johnson, O. N. *Essentials of Dental Radiography for Dental Assistants and Hygienists*. 4th ed. Norwalk, Conn.: Appleton & Lange, 1990.

Eastman Kodak Company. *X-Rays in Dentistry*. Rochester, N.Y.: Radiology Markets Division, 1985.

Frommer, H. H. *Radiology for Dental Auxiliaries*. 4th ed. St. Louis: C. V. Mosby Co., 1987.

Section 4

Examination

In a few words, phrases, or sentences, answer the following questions. Use a separate sheet of paper.

1. List four requirements for the design of a darkroom.
2. What are the two types of lights used in a darkroom?
3. What is a safelight?
4. List two types of filters used in safelights, and specify when each type should be used.
5. List two ways to check a darkroom for light leaks.
6. List five parts of a developing tank.
7. How is the temperature of the processing chemicals maintained?
8. List two advantages of automatic processors.
9. How does an automatic processor develop films in 5 minutes?
10. List and describe the function of three darkroom accessories.
11. List the chemicals in the developer, and give the action of each.
12. List the chemicals in the fixer, and give the action of each.
13. Describe the controlled time-temperature method of processing.
14. If the temperature of the developer is 70°F, give the times films should be left in:
    a. Developer
    b. Fixer
15. Describe the use of the embossed dot on the film.
16. a. What are the two basic components of radiographic film?
    b. List the components and give the purpose of each.
17. What determines the speed of the film?
18. Define and compare non-screen and screen films.
19. List the events that take place in the film emulsion during the exposure and processing of the film.
20. Define radiographic density, contrast, and detail.
21. List four quality-assurance procedures that relate to film processing.

Intraoral Radiographic Techniques

Exposure of intraoral radiographs is one of the most important procedures performed by the dental radiographer. Modern dentistry has become increasingly dependent on interpretations made from radiographs. Supported by the principles of shadow casting, this section graphically demonstrates the most common intraoral projections.

OBJECTIVES

1. To compare intraoral and extraoral radiographic techniques.
2. To discuss the structures demonstrated on periapical and bitewing radiographs.
3. To list and discuss the five principles of shadow casting.
4. To describe how the vertical and horizontal angulation is adjusted for intraoral radiographic procedures.
5. To discuss the reasons that the paralleling technique was developed.
6. To list and discuss the four rules of procedure for the Stabe paralleling technique.
7. To identify advantages of the Precision paralleling technique.
8. To discuss how the vertical angulation is established in the bisecting-the-angle technique.
9. To list and discuss the four rules of procedure for the bisecting-the-angle technique.
10. To discuss the advantages and disadvantages of the paralleling and bisecting-the-angle techniques.
11. To discuss packet placement and cone angulations used to obtain premolar and molar radiographs.
12. To recognize common errors in periapical technique.

INTRODUCTION

Intraoral radiography is accomplished by placing the film packet inside the patient's mouth and directing x rays from outside the mouth through the teeth and onto the film. This is distinct from extraoral radiography, in which both the x-ray source and the film are outside the mouth. Extraoral techniques are discussed in Section 6. Intraoral radiographs are characterized by images with excellent detail. The fine detail is required for the diagnosis of dental diseases such as caries and periodontal disease. The use of non-screen film in the dental packets provides the required detail.

TYPES OF PROJECTIONS

Periapical and bitewing radiographs are intraoral projections routinely obtained in the dental office. A *periapical* film shows the entire tooth and the structures around the root apex and is used to detect periapical infections. The *bitewing* radiograph demonstrates the crowns of the maxillary and mandibular teeth along with the bony crests of the alveolar ridges. The bitewing film is used to detect interproximal caries and periodontal disease.

Two other intraoral projections also widely used are the occlusal and the third molar disto-oblique. An *occlusal* projection is used as a survey film for larger areas of the jaw. The *third molar disto-oblique* radiograph is used to visualize third molars that are

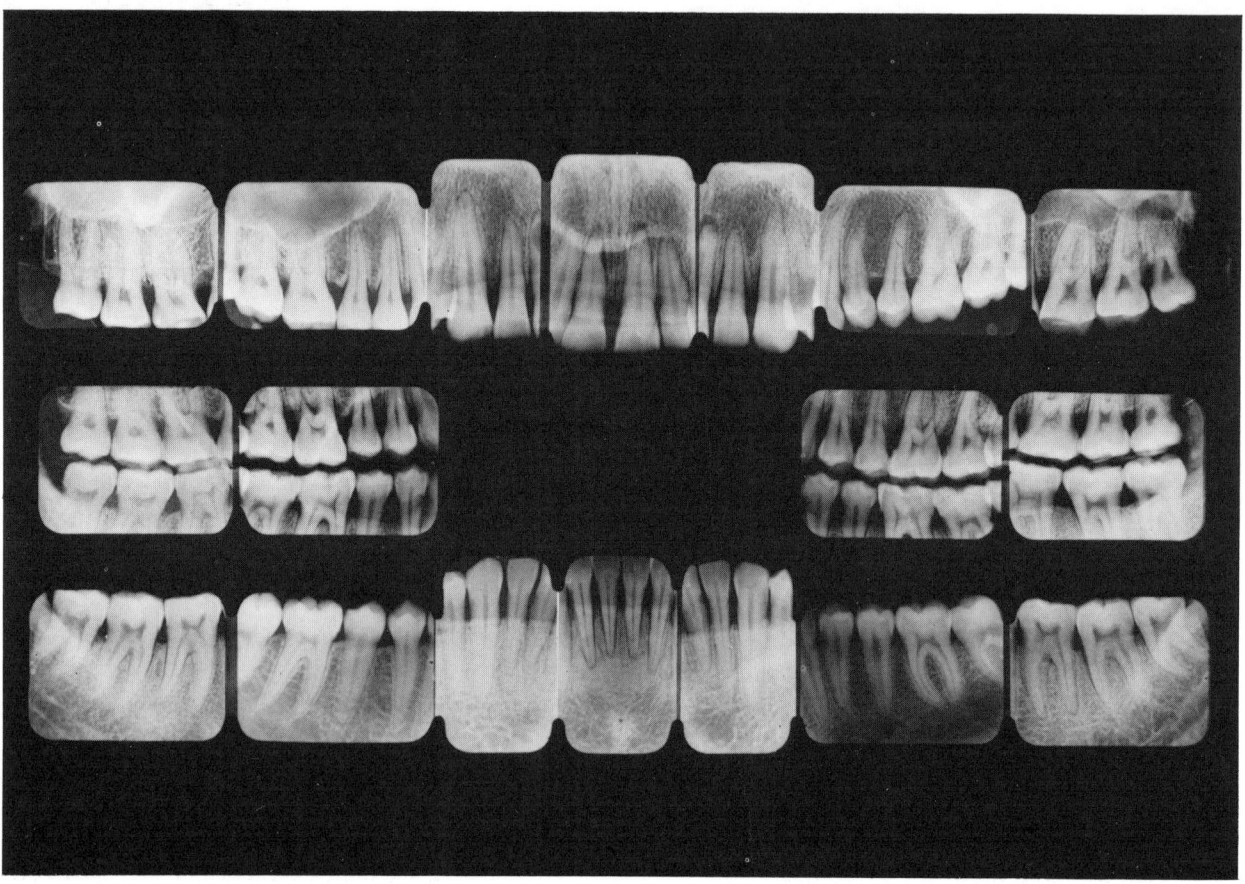

Fig. 1, V-5 Full series of intraoral radiographs.

not completely demonstrated on the usual molar projections.

Individual periapical and bitewing radiographs are often used individually for diagnostic purposes or together to form a "full series" of a patient. For this manual 14 periapical and 4 bitewing projections are considered a full series. The full series adequately shows all areas of the adult jaws and teeth (Fig. 1, V-5).

SHADOW CASTING

The accuracy of the image obtained using any radiographic technique is dependent on adherence to the five principles of shadow casting.

The Five Principles of Shadow Casting

Principle 1. *X rays should be emitted from as small a point source of radiation as possible.* The use of a smaller focal spot on the target of the anode in the tubehead results in more parallel x rays. X rays that are parallel cause the x-ray beam to be more consis-

tent, resulting in film images with better detail. In dental x-ray machines the focal spot size is established by the manufacturer and cannot be changed by the operator. Many medical machines do provide the operator a choice of focal spot size.

Principle 2. *The distance from the x-ray source (focal spot) to the object (tooth) should be as long as possible* (Fig. 2, V-5). The use of longer cones on dental machines is an example of using a longer source-to-object distance. Because less divergent x rays are used to produce the image, the edges of the teeth appear sharper and the size of the teeth more realistic (less magnified).

Principle 3. *The distance from the object (tooth) to the film should be as short as possible* (Fig. 3, V-5). As the film is placed closer to the teeth, there is less distance present to blur or enlarge the shadow. A shorter distance between object and film decreases magnification and improves the sharpness of the images.

Principle 4. *The object (tooth) and the film should be parallel to each other* (Fig. 4, V-5). By arranging the film packet parallel to the long axis of the tooth, less distortion of the image is seen.

Principle 5. *The x-ray beam should be directed at a right angle to the film and the tooth* (Fig. 4, V-5). When the film is placed parallel with the tooth, distortion is reduced by directing the x-ray beam at right angles to both the teeth and the film. If the beam is tilted, the tooth images are distorted.

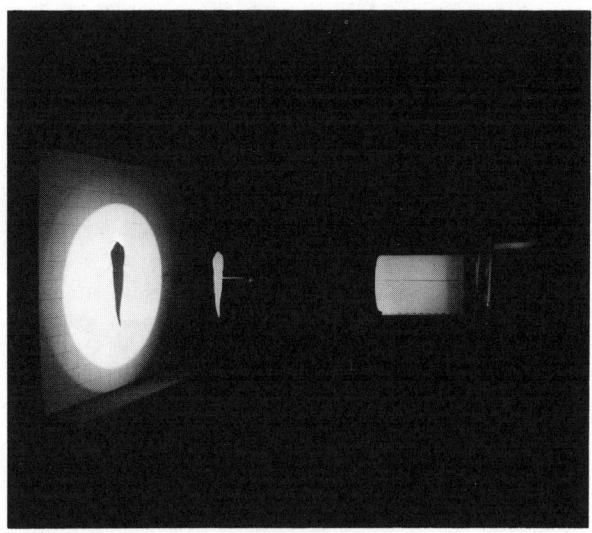

Fig. 2, V-5 Shadow-casting Principle 2.
A. Short x-ray source-to-tooth distance results in enlarged tooth image (increased magnification).

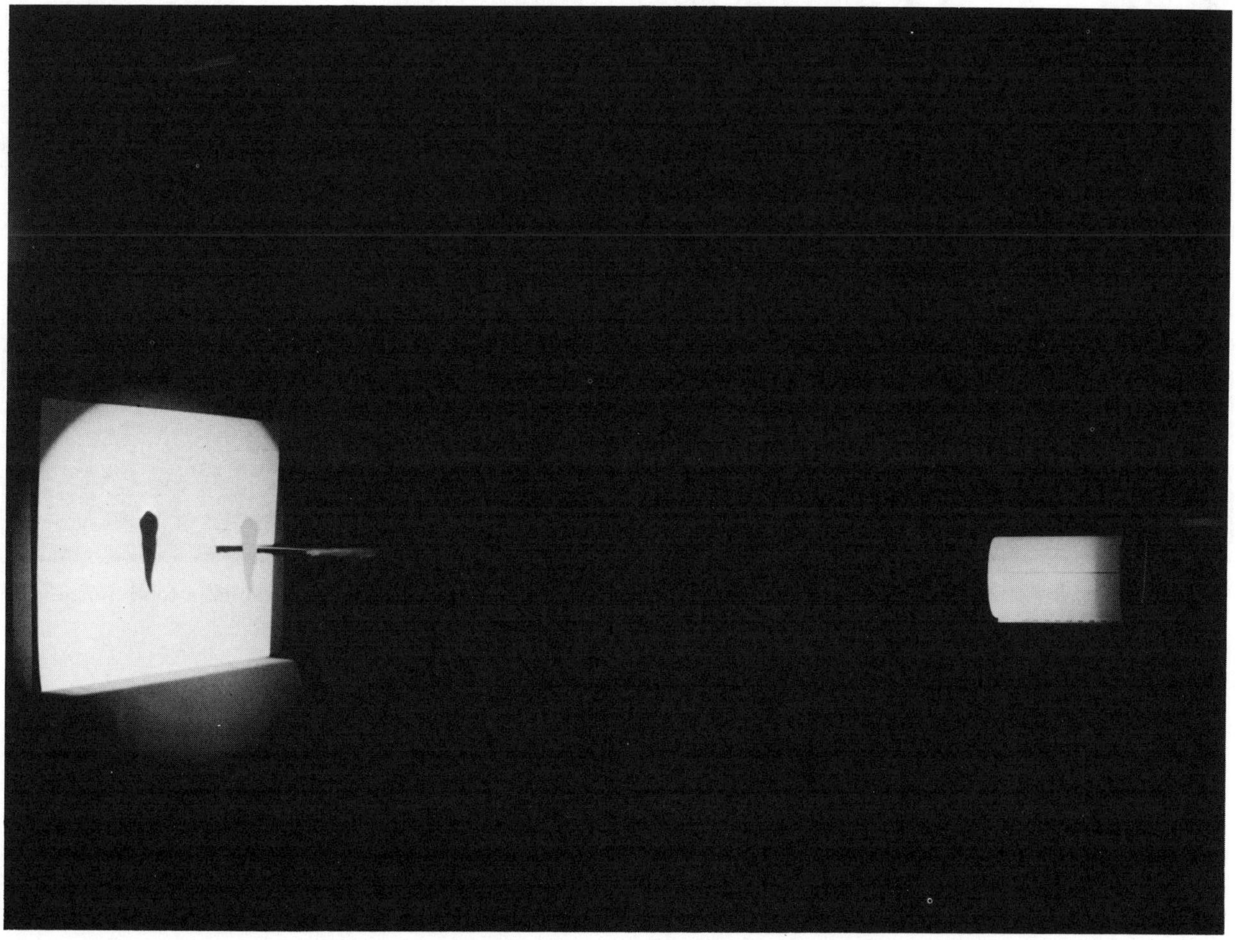

B. Long x-ray source-to-tooth distance results in tooth image with less magnification.

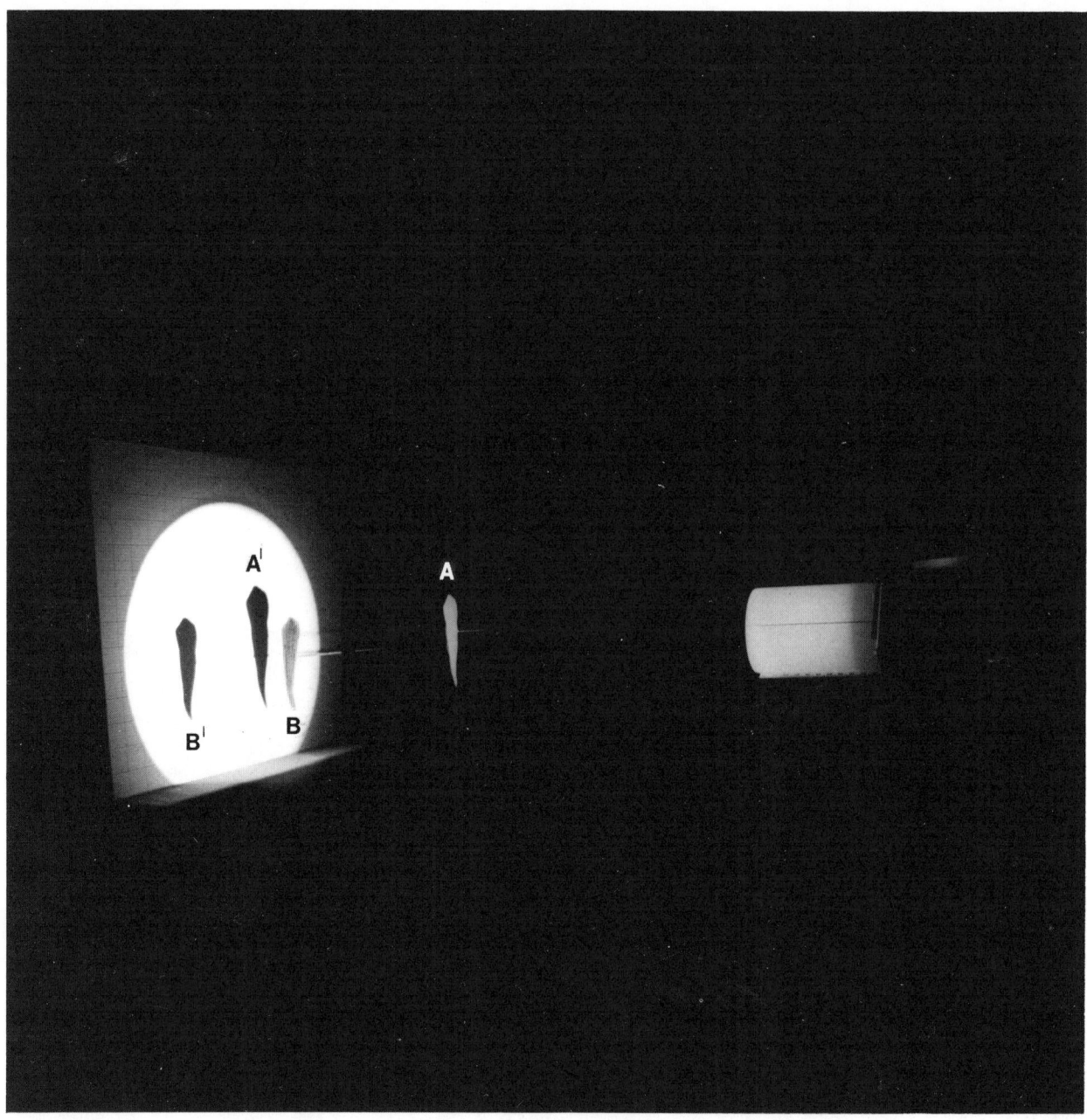

Fig. 3, V-5 Shadow-casting Principle 3.
Tooth farther from film (A) results in enlarged tooth image (A').

Tooth closer to film (B) results in tooth image with less magnification (B').

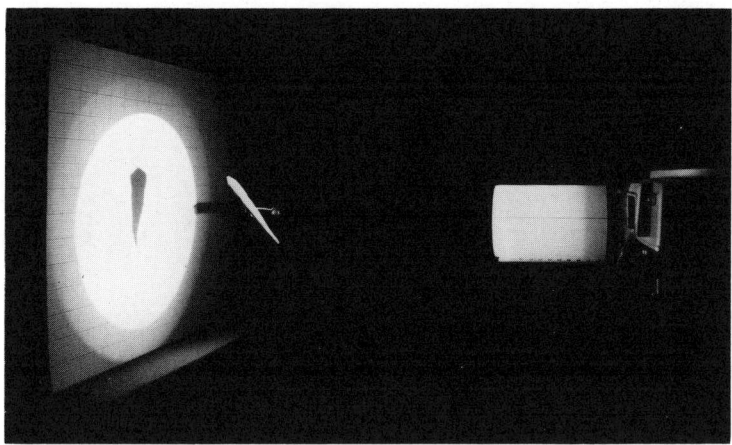

Fig. 4, V-5 Shadow-casting Principles 4 and 5.

   A. Tooth not parallel to film results in distorted tooth image.

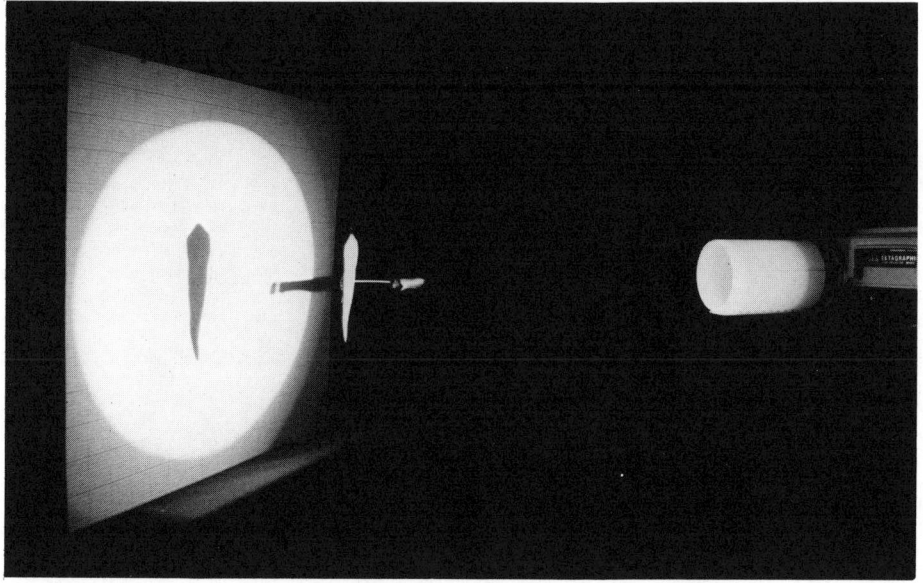

   B. X-ray source not perpendicular to tooth and film, resulting in distorted film image.

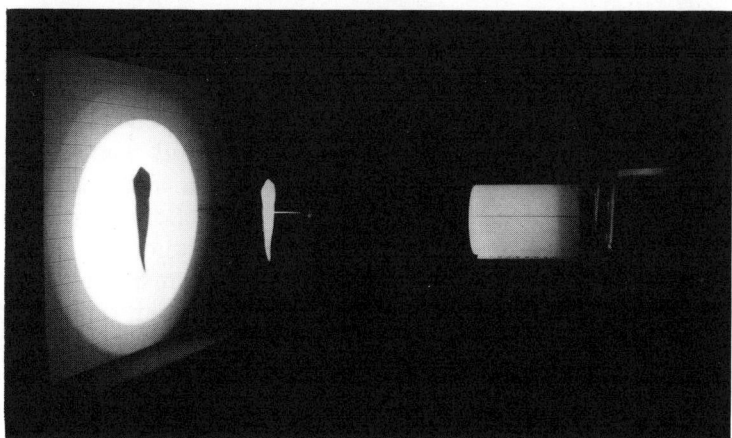

C. Tooth parallel to film and x-ray beam are perpendicular.

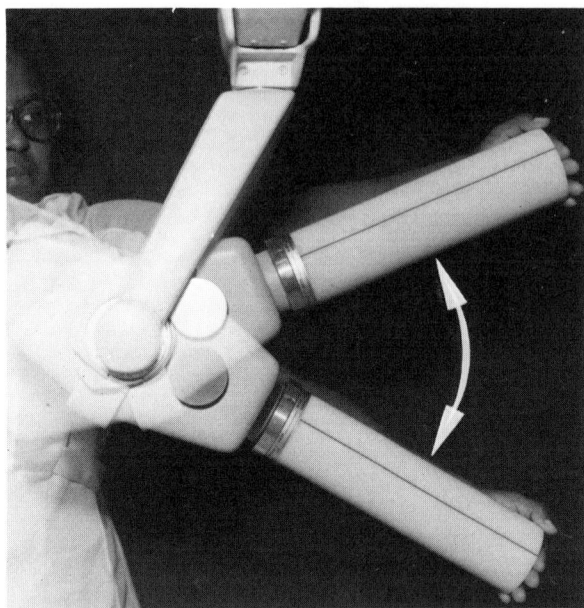

Fig. 5, V-5 Basic cone alignments.
A. Vertical angulation.

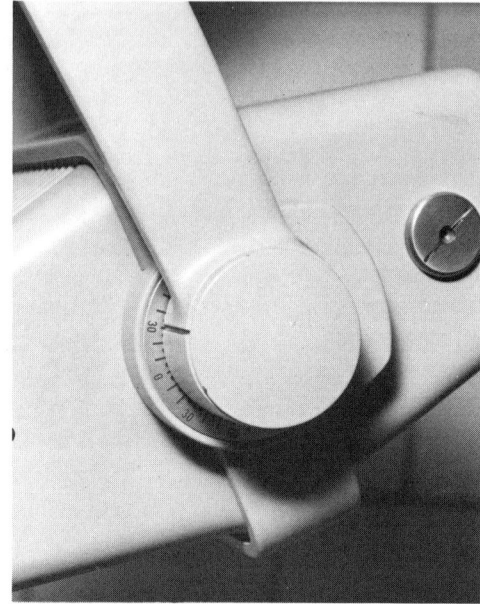

B. Dial on tubehead indicating vertical angulation in degrees.

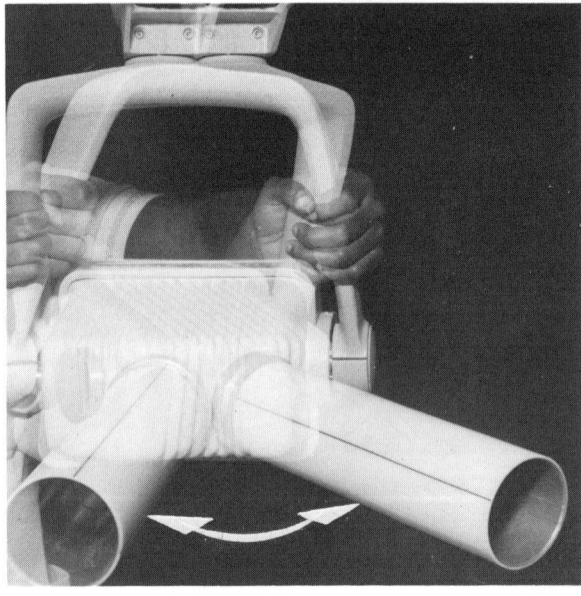

C. Horizontal angulation.

BASIC CONE ANGULATIONS

Two angulations of the cone and tubehead established while taking intraoral radiographs are vertical and horizontal. *Vertical angulation* is established by rotating the extension cone in an upward-and-downward motion. Notice that changes in vertical angulation can be measured in degrees as registered on a dial located on the side of the dental x-ray tubehead. For the paralleling method the vertical angulation used is determined by the planes of the teeth

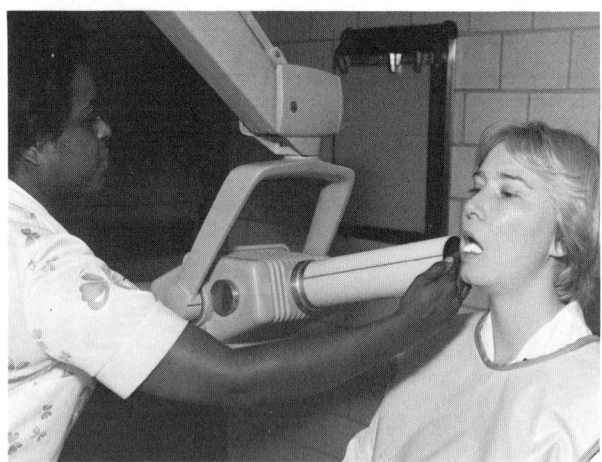

Fig. 6, V-5 Hand over end of cone to protect patient.

and film. For the bisecting-the-angle method an established angle is used for each projection (Fig. 5A, B, V-5).

Horizontal angulation is established by placing the hands on both sides of the tubehead and rotating the dental cone and tubehead in a side-to-side motion. Setting the correct horizontal angulation is accomplished by judging the direction required to direct the x-ray beam through the interproximal spaces of the teeth and aligning the cone accordingly (Fig. 5C, V-5). When moving the cone next to the face of the patient, it is helpful if the operator places a hand over the open end of the cone. This prevents accidentally jarring the patient with the edge of the cone (Fig. 6, V-5).

PERIAPICAL TECHNIQUES

The two most commonly used methods for obtaining periapical radiographs are the paralleling and bisecting-the-angle techniques.

PARALLELING TECHNIQUE

The paralleling technique of periapical radiography was introduced in 1947 by McCormack in order to provide radiographs of the teeth with a minimum of image distortion and a minimum of superimposition of adjacent structures. It is also referred to as the *right-angle method* and the *long-cone technique*. The paralleling technique is generally preferred for periapical radiography today because it more closely follows the principles of shadow casting than the bisecting-the-angle method.

The paralleling technique is based on the placement of the film packet with its long axis parallel to the long axis of the teeth (Fig. 7, V-5). In order to carry out this procedure the film must be positioned some distance away from the lingual sides of the teeth. Because this violates the principle that the object-to-film distance should be as short as possible, a longer cone (16-in.) is used. The longer focal spot-to-tooth distance resulting from the use of the long cone corrects for the space between the teeth and the film, so that resulting images are clearly defined and only slightly magnified.

After placing the film parallel to the teeth, the vertical angulation is established by directing the x-ray beam at right angles to the film. Four rules of procedure are to be followed when employing the paralleling technique. The operator should accomplish each film in the following step-by-step fashion to achieve good results: packet placement, vertical angulation, horizontal angulation, and centering of the exposure field.

Film holders are used to position the film packet in the required locations. A variety of devices are available for this purpose, including the Precision Instruments (Isaac Masel Co., Philadelphia PA), the Rinn Instruments (Rinn Corp., Elgin, IL), and the Stabe holder (Greene Dental Products, Inc., San Fernando, CA). In this manual only the Stabe holder and Precision Instruments are illustrated, but the same principles apply to the other holders.

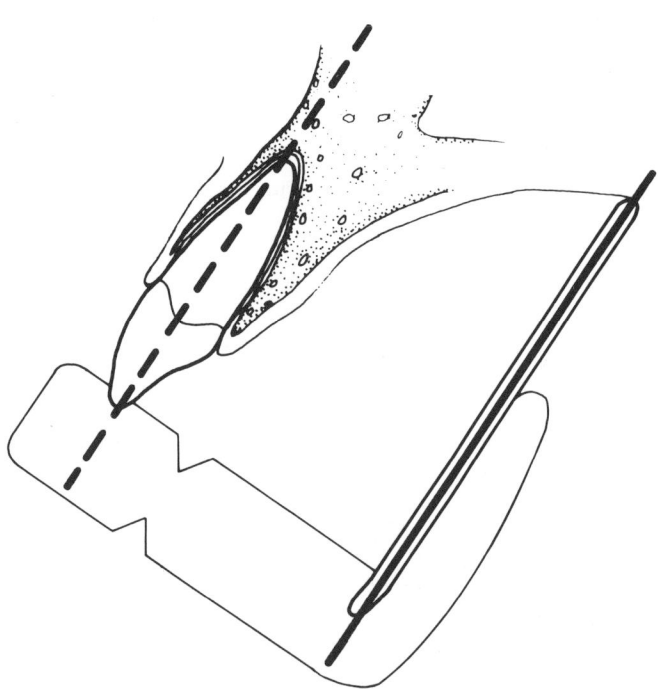

Fig. 7, V-5 Principles of paralleling technique. Packet placed parallel to long axis of tooth. (From *Intraoral Radiography: The Paralleling Technique*, by Cy Whaley [Chapel Hill, N.C.: University of North Carolina, 1977])

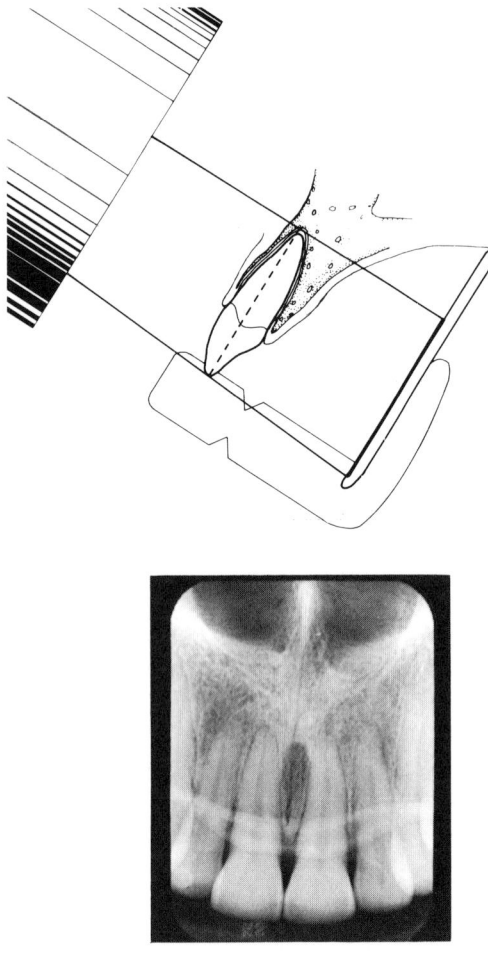

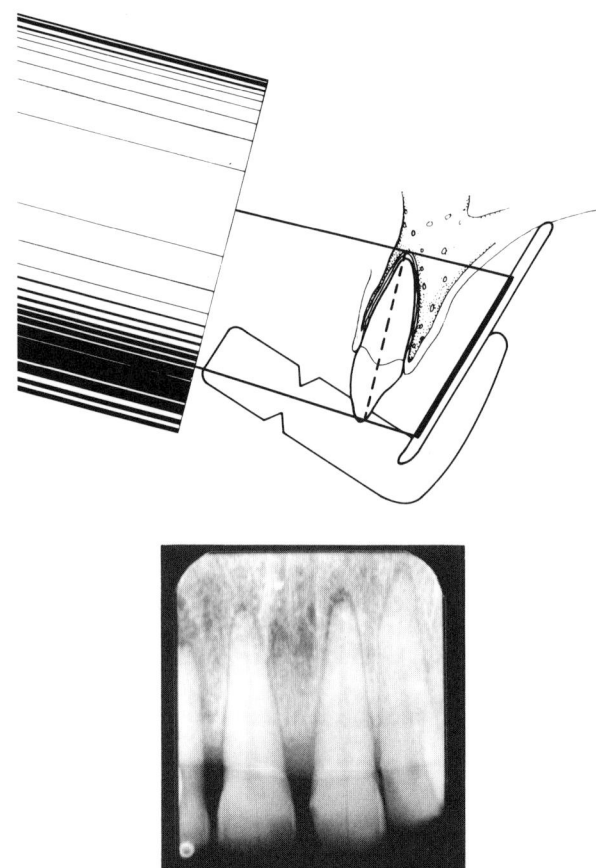

Fig. 8, V-5 Rule 1: Packet placement.
A. Packet placed parallel to long axis of tooth.
B. Resulting radiograph. (From *Intraoral Radiography: The Paralleling Technique*, by Cy Whaley [Chapel Hill, N.C.: University of North Carolina, 1977])

Fig. 9, V-5 Incorrect packet placement.
A. Tooth and film planes not parallel.
B. Resulting radiograph. (From *Intraoral Radiography: The Paralleling Technique*, by Cy Whaley [Chapel Hill, N.C.: University of North Carolina, 1977])

Four Rules of Procedure for the Paralleling Technique

Rule 1. *Packet Placement: Place the film parallel to the long axis of the teeth.* In order to achieve correct packet placement, the film must be positioned within the oral cavity so that the long axis of the entire tooth and that of the film packet are parallel to each other. In the maxillary region, the top edge of the film is the same distance from the apex (root tip) of the tooth as the bottom edge of the film is from the occlusal surface of the tooth. Visualization of this relationship prior to making an exposure is essential. Figure 8A, V-5 with corresponding radiograph B, illustrates correct packet placement for a maxillary central incisor projection. This illustration shows a Stabe film holder being used and demonstrates how the teeth being radiographed occlude onto a designated bite area of the Stabe. For this projection, notice how the film is forced away from the tooth, establishing the correct parallel relationship. Arranging for the biting surfaces of the teeth being radiographed to touch the proper place on the Stabe is as important as actually seeing the parallel relationship between the film plane and the tooth plane.

Figures 9A and B, V-5 illustrate incorrect packet placement and radiograph resulting from failure to place the film packet parallel to the teeth. Notice the elongated teeth. By comparison, the correctly exposed radiograph in Figure 8B, V-5 demonstrates the tooth in correct proportions. Images free from distortion are essential for accurate diagnosis and cannot be obtained without correct placement of the film.

Rule 2. *Vertical Angulation: Align the x-ray cone at a right angle to the film surface.* This rule follows shadow-casting Principle 4, and its use eliminates distortion of the tooth images. Notice in Figure 10, V-5 that the tooth and film are parallel and the x-ray cone is aligned perpendicular to the tooth and the film. Imagine one x ray, often referred to as the central ray, exiting from the center of the cone and forming a perfect "T" with the planes of the long axis of the tooth and film. This "T" relationship is included in these illustrations to assist in visualizing and understanding the proper relationship between the film and the x-ray cone. Another method one might use when establishing the vertical angulation is to visualize the base of the Stabe and the bottom of the cone as two independent straight lines. By bringing them together as one line, the central ray will be directed at a right angle to the film plane. Either method works when following Rule 2. Figures 11A, B and 12A, B, V-5 are provided to illustrate the appearance of incorrect vertical angulation. These appearances should be studied in detail so that such situations are corrected as they occur.

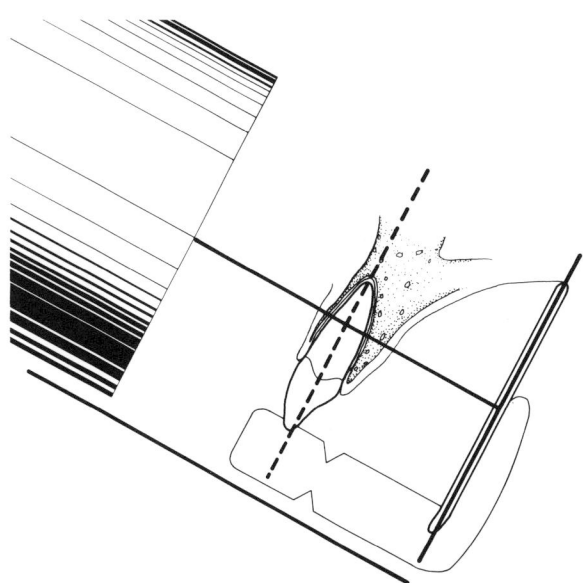

Fig. 10, V-5 Rule 2: Vertical angulation. Direct x rays at a right angle to tooth and film. (From *Intraoral Radiography: The Paralleling Technique,* by Cy Whaley [Chapel Hill, N.C.: University of North Carolina, 1977])

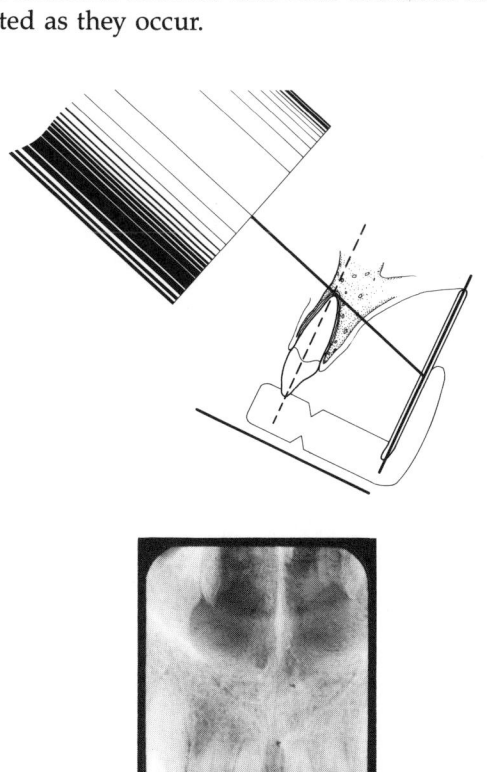

Fig. 11, V-5 Incorrect vertical angulation.
    A. Vertical angle too steep.
    B. Resulting radiograph. (From *Intraoral Radiography: The Paralleling Technique,* by Cy Whaley [Chapel Hill, N.C.: University of North Carolina, 1977])

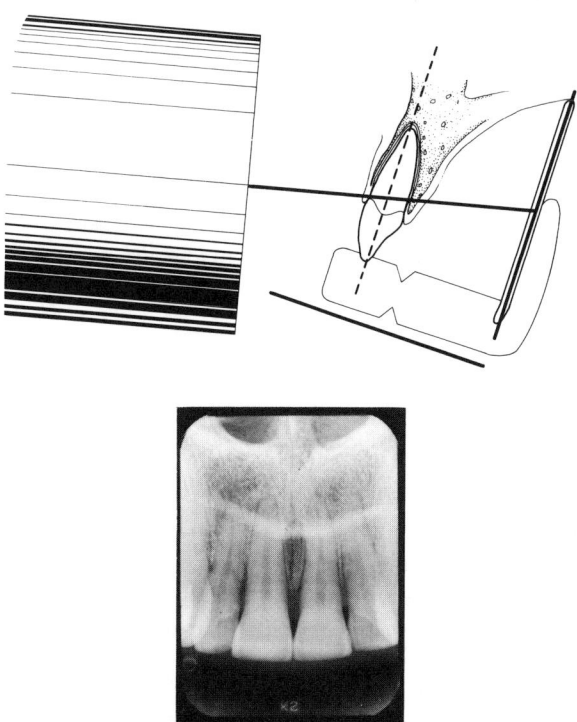

Fig. 12, V-5 Incorrect vertical angulation.
    A. Vertical angle too flat.
    B. Resulting radiograph. (From *Intraoral Radiography: The Paralleling Technique,* by Cy Whaley [Chapel Hill, N.C.: University of North Carolina, 1977]

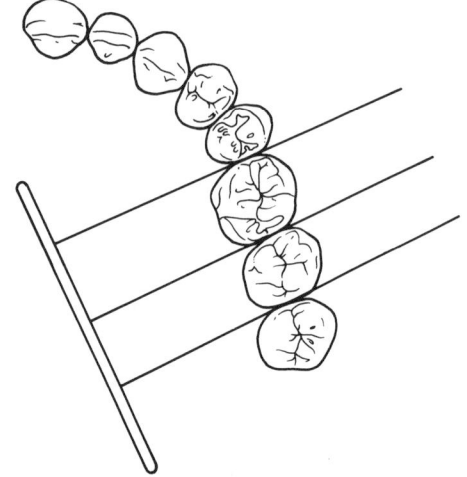

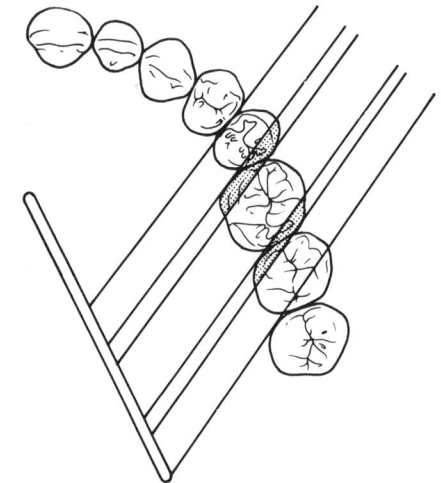

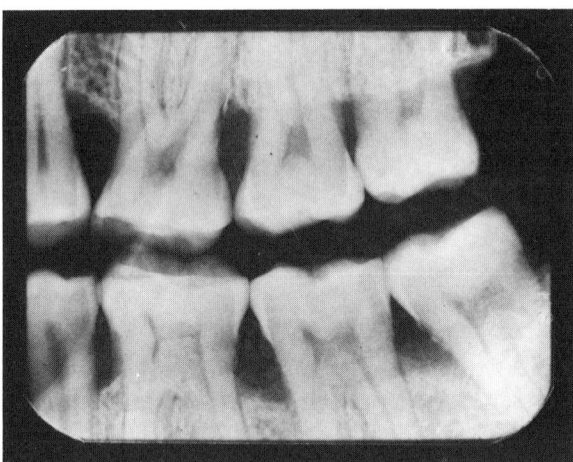

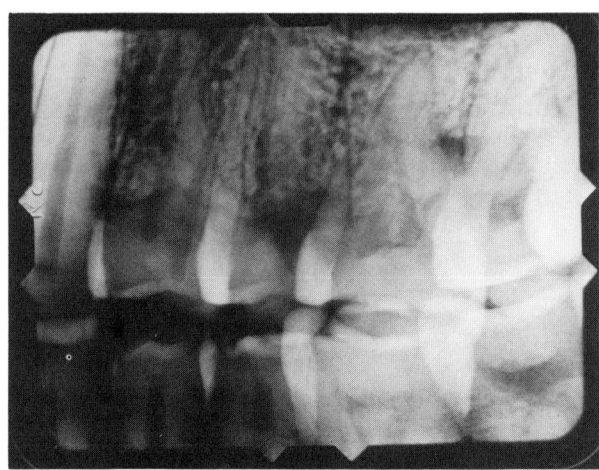

Fig. 13, V-5 Rule 3: Horizontal angulation.
A. Direct x rays through interproximal spaces.
B. Resulting radiograph. (From *Intraoral Radiography: The Paralleling Technique*, by Cy Whaley [Chapel Hill, N.C.: University of North Carolina, 1977])

Fig. 14, V-5 Incorrect horizontal angulation.
A. Incorrect alignment of x-ray beam.
B. Resulting radiograph. (From *Intraoral Radiography: The Paralleling Technique*, by Cy Whaley [Chapel Hill, N.C.: University of North Carolina, 1977])

Rule 3. *Horizontal Angulation: Direct the x-ray beam through the spaces between the teeth.* Figure 13A, B, V-5 demonstrates the principle of directing the x rays through the interproximal spaces, those spaces between the teeth. The diagnosis of caries is dependent on being able to see the mesial and distal surfaces of the teeth without overlapping of the adjacent tooth. After completing packet placement and verti-

cal angulation, the operator should stand behind the tubehead and align the cone, directing the central ray through the interproximal surfaces of interest. Figure 14A, V-5 illustrates the incorrect alignment of the x-ray beam. Also shown is the appearance of overlapped interproximal spaces on a bitewing projection (Fig. 14B, V-5).

Rule 4. *Centering the exposure field on the film: Cover the film packet with the x-ray beam.* It is important that the x-ray beam cover the film packet. Failure to cover it results in unexposed, clear areas on the film, called *cone cuts*. Even when the cone is properly positioned in the vertical and horizontal planes, it can be out of position, causing some of the film to be missed by the x-ray beam. To prevent cone cuts, the cone should be aligned so that its open end is centered over the film packet. After establishing the vertical and horizontal angulations, minor changes in cone position are made by standing behind the tubehead and "sighting" down the sides of the cone. The operator should visualize that the x-ray beam will cover the four sides of the film (Fig. 15A, B, V-5). The broken-line circle area demonstrates where the cone should be for a maxillary premolar projection, whereas the dark circle area indicates the location of the cone during the exposure of the incorrect radiograph.

THE MANDIBULAR PREMOLAR AND MOLAR PROJECTIONS. Because of the anatomy of the floor of the mouth, enough space is available for the film packet to be placed close to the teeth *and* also to be parallel to the teeth. This is in contrast to the procedure used in the mandibular anterior and all maxillary projections, where, because of the shape of the alveolar crest and palate, the film packet must be moved away from the teeth to achieve a parallel relationship. Figure 16, V-5 illustrates packet placement for the mandibular posterior teeth. Notice that *the end section of the Stabe is removed to permit correct placement as well as to avoid impingement on the patient's cheek.*

INDIVIDUAL PROJECTIONS. Figures 17-24, V-5 illustrate the packet placement, vertical and horizontal cone angulations, and centering of the exposure field for the eight standard projections using the paralleling technique. The Stabe holder is used, but the same principles apply with other holders. No. 1 size films are used for the four lateral incisor-canine radiographs and the mandibular central incisor radiograph. No. 2 size films are used for the maxillary central incisor projection and all posterior periapical films.

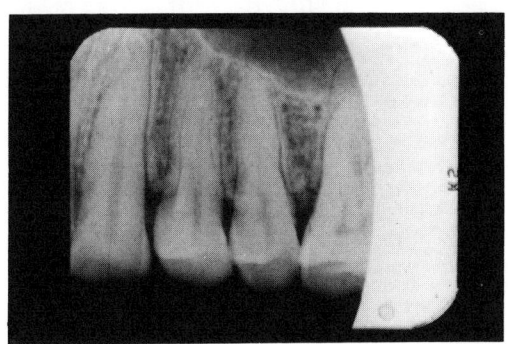

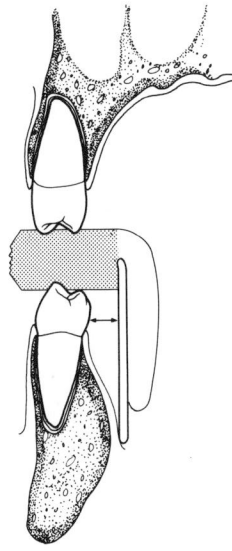

Fig. 15, V-5 Rule 4: Centering of exposure field.
A. Incorrect and correct centering of cone.
B. Resulting radiograph of incorrect centering of cone. (From *Intraoral Radiography: The Paralleling Technique,* by Cy Whaley [Chapel Hill, N.C.: University of North Carolina, 1977])

Fig. 16, V-5 Packet placement for mandibular premolar and molar projections.

STABE PARALLELING TECHNIQUE
Maxillary Central Incisor

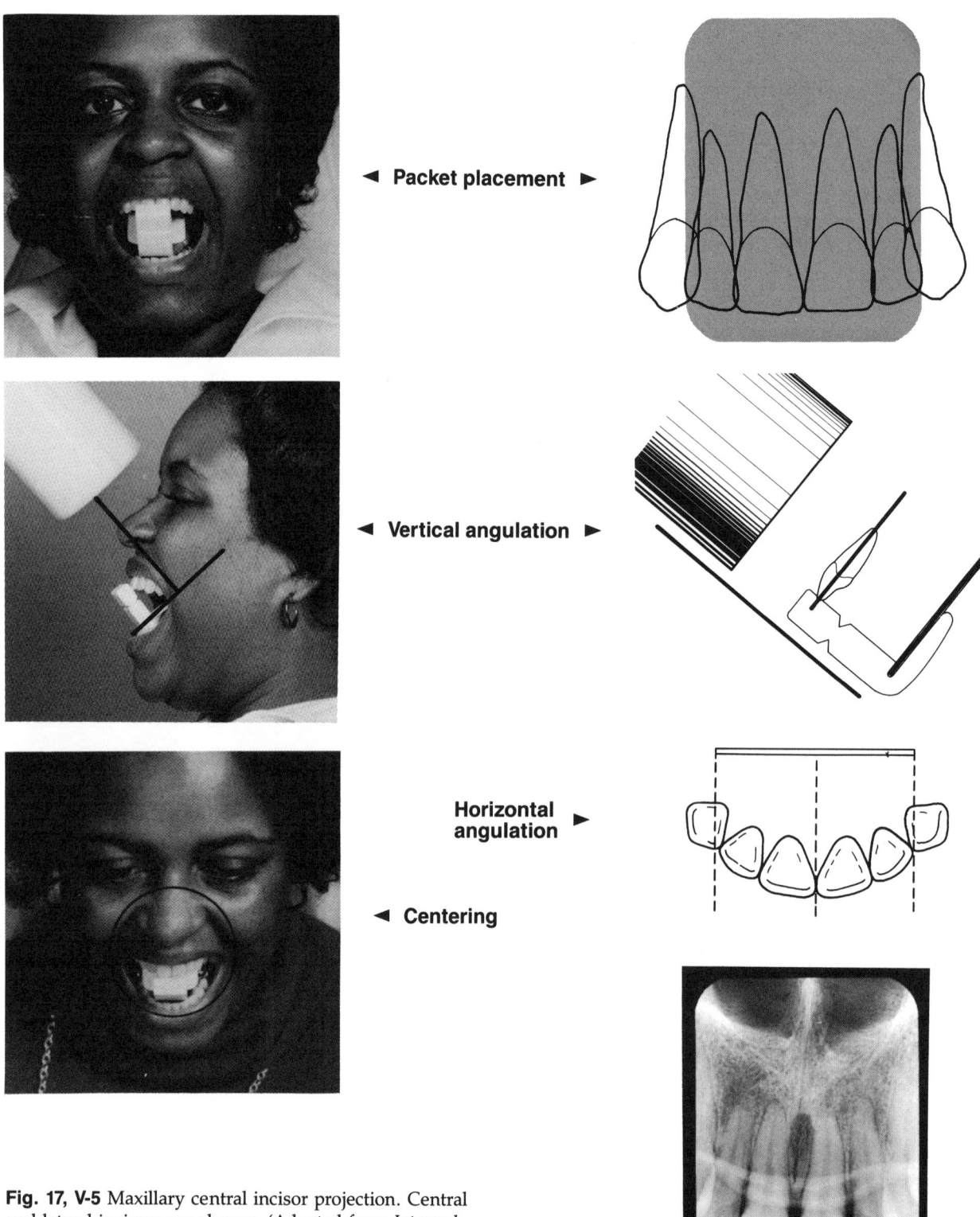

◀ **Packet placement** ▶

◀ **Vertical angulation** ▶

Horizontal angulation ▶

◀ **Centering**

Fig. 17, V-5 Maxillary central incisor projection. Central and lateral incisors are shown. (Adapted from *Intraoral Radiography: The Paralleling Technique*, by Cy Whaley [Chapel Hill, N.C.: University of North Carolina, 1977])

STABE PARALLELING TECHNIQUE
Maxillary Lateral Incisor—Canine

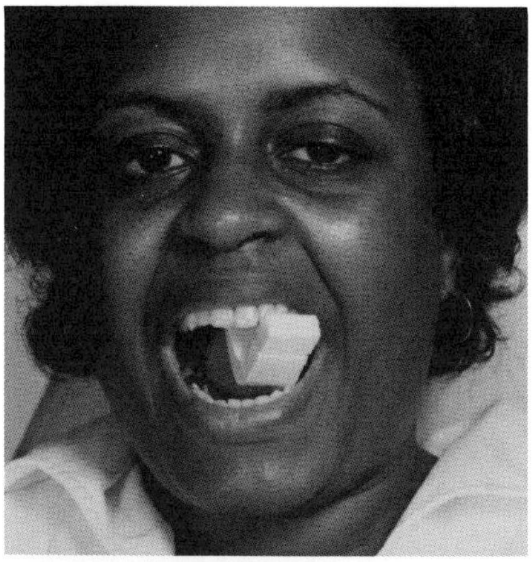

◄ **Packet placement** ►

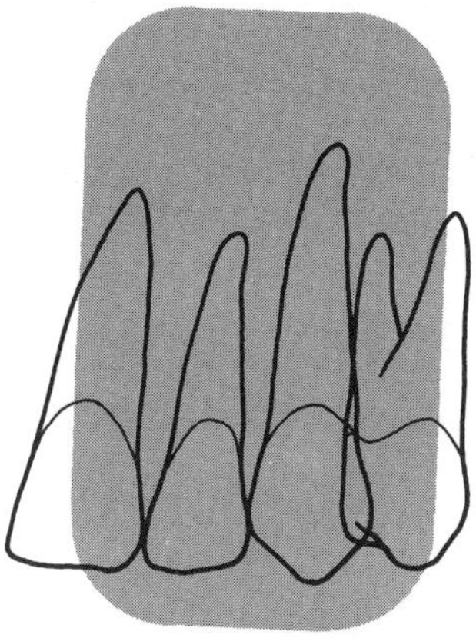

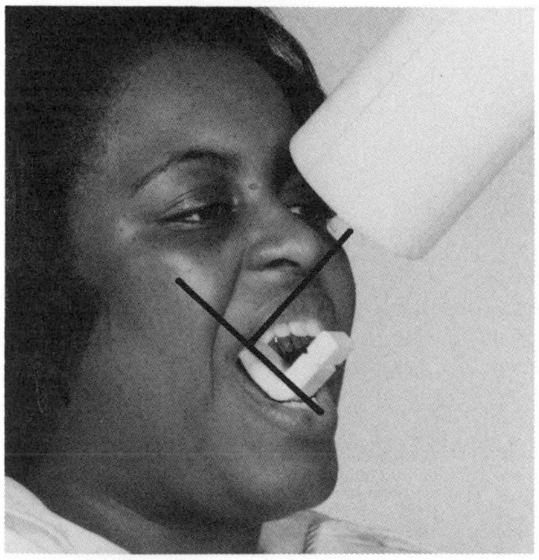

◄ **Vertical angulation** ►

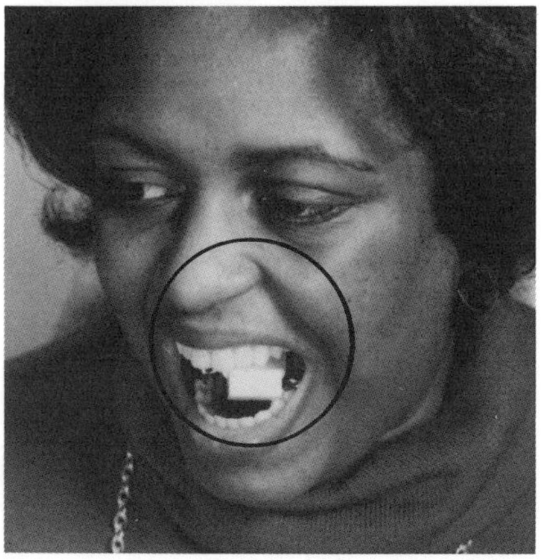

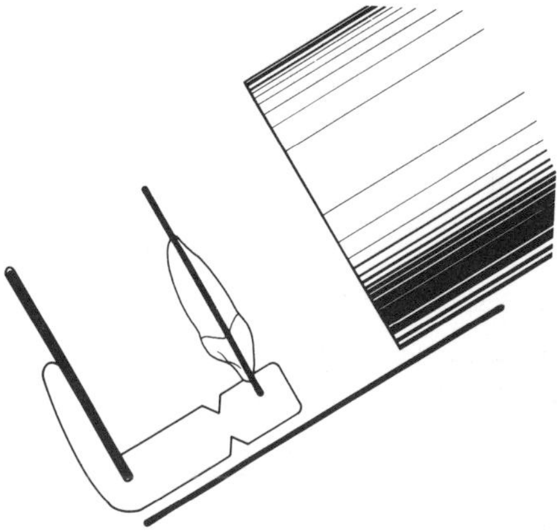

Horizontal angulation ►

◄ **Centering**

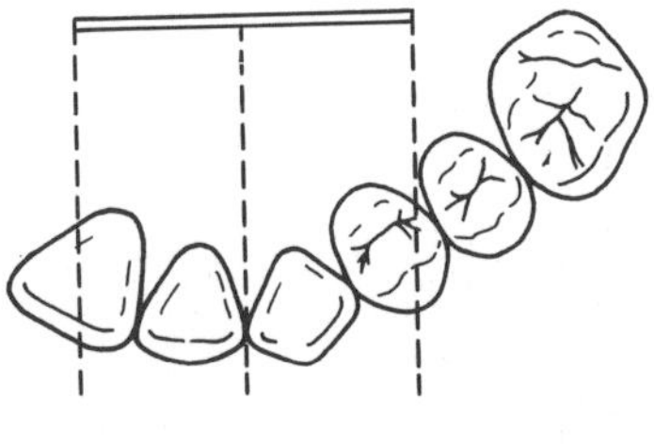

Fig. 18, V-5 Maxillary lateral incisor-canine projection. Lateral incisor and canine are shown. (Adapted from *Intraoral Radiography: The Paralleling Technique*, by Cy Whaley [Chapel Hill, N.C.: University of North Carolina, 1977])

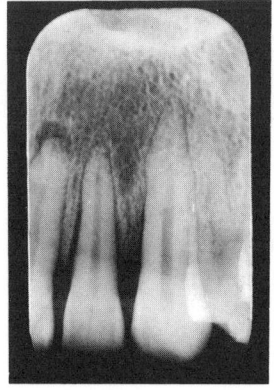

STABE PARALLELING TECHNIQUE
Maxillary Premolar

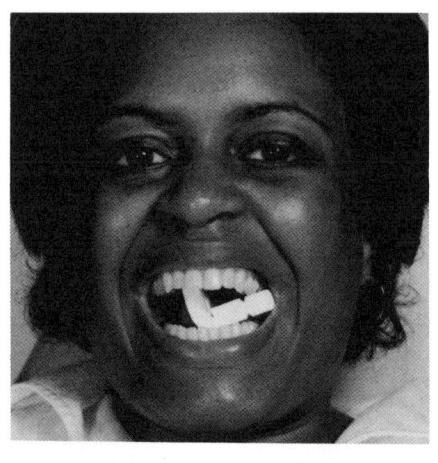

◀ **Packet placement** ▶

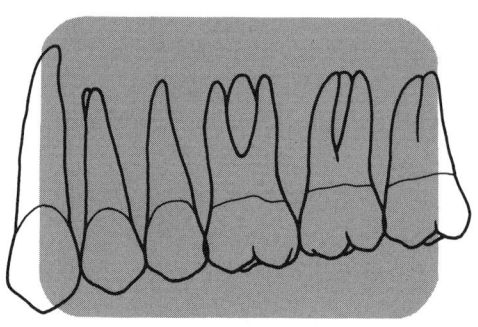

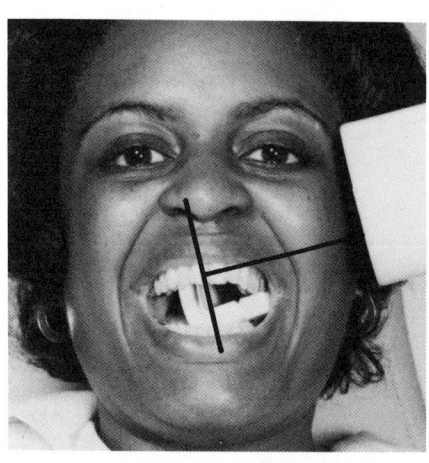

◀ **Vertical angulation** ▶

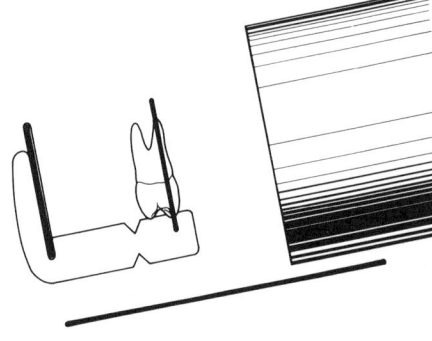

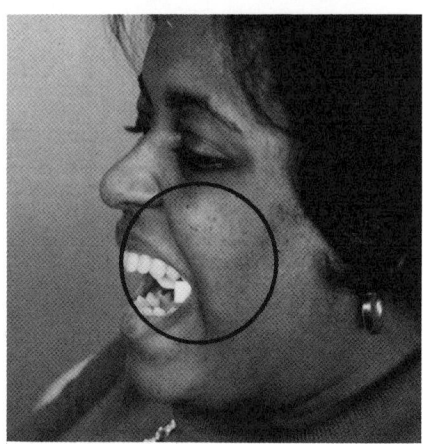

Horizontal angulation ▶

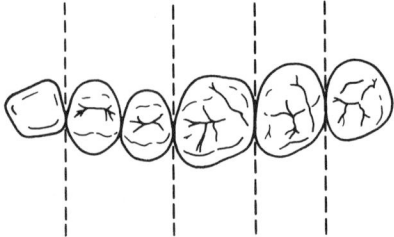

◀ **Centering**

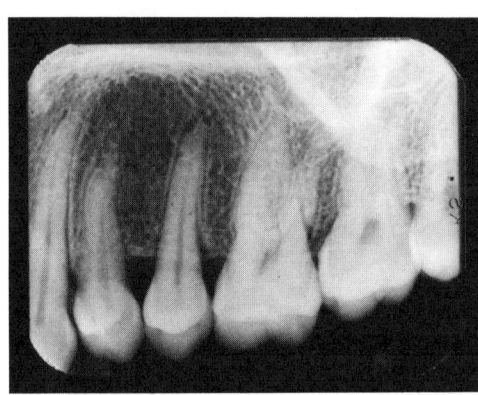

Fig. 19, V-5 Maxillary premolar projection. Distal half of canine, both premolars and first molar are shown. (Adapted from *Intraoral Radiography: The Paralleling Technique,* by Cy Whaley [Chapel Hill, N.C.: University of North Carolina, 1977])

90

STABE PARALLELING TECHNIQUE
Maxillary Molar

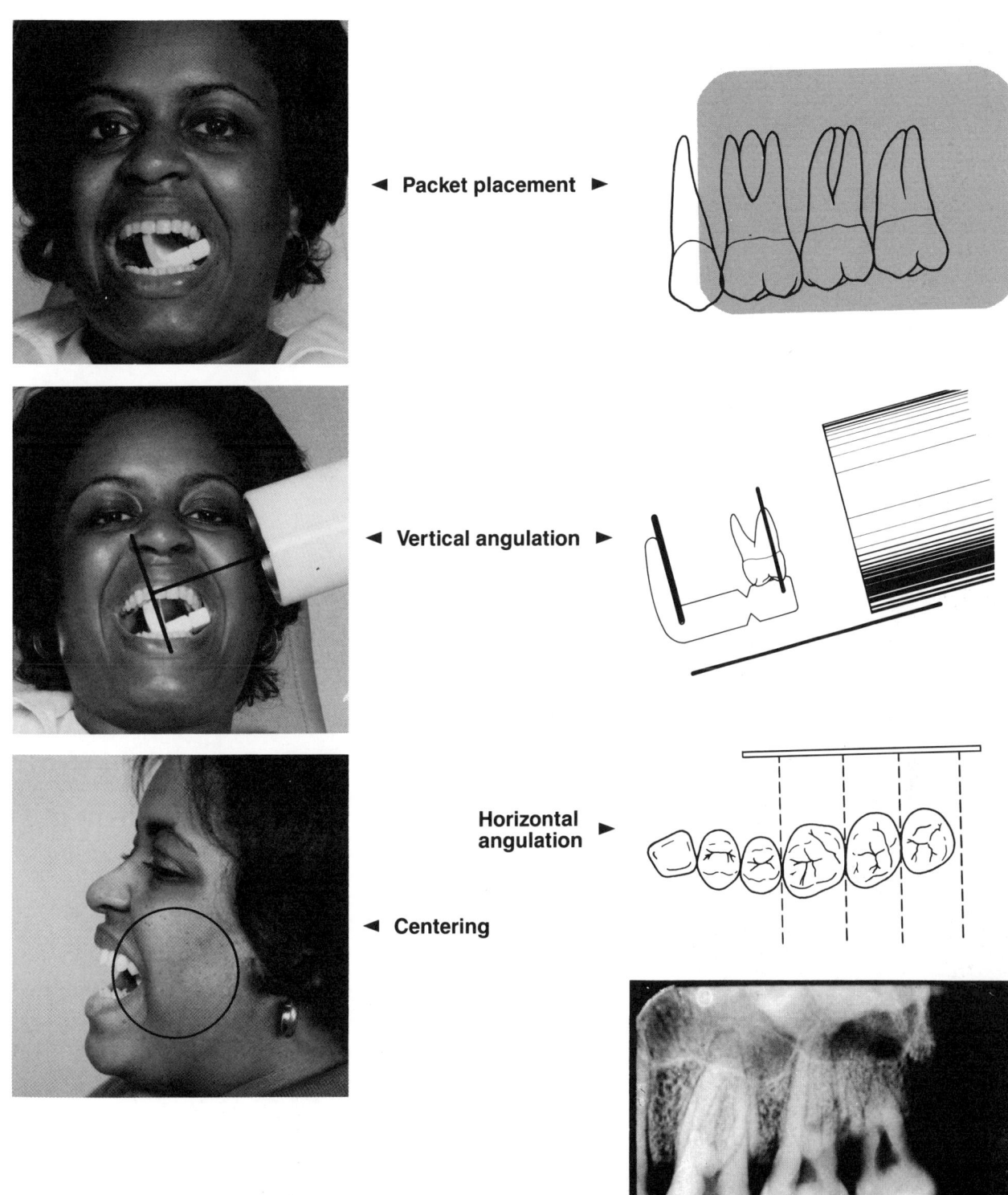

◄ **Packet placement** ►

◄ **Vertical angulation** ►

Horizontal angulation ►

◄ **Centering**

Fig. 20, V-5 Maxillary molar projection. First, second, and third molars are shown. (Adapted from *Intraoral Radiography: The Paralleling Technique*, by Cy Whaley [Chapel Hill, N.C.: University of North Carolina, 1977])

STABE PARALLELING TECHNIQUE
Mandibular Central Incisor

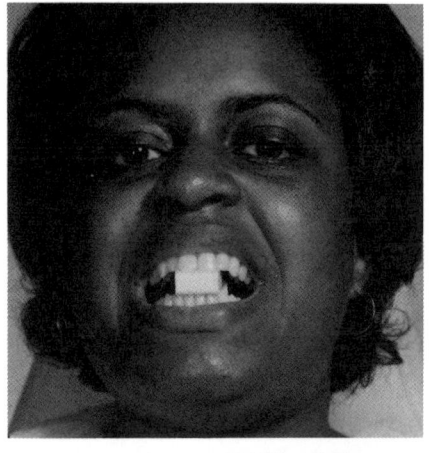

◄ **Packet placement** ►

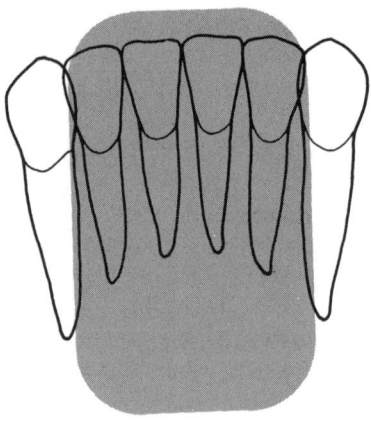

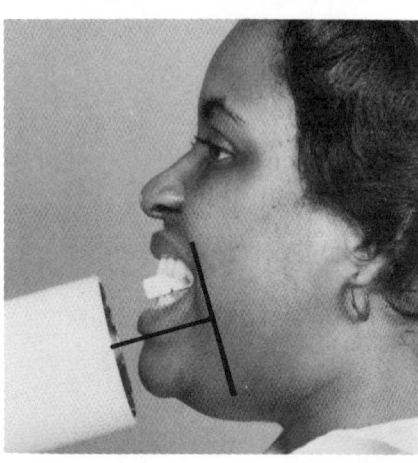

◄ **Vertical angulation** ►

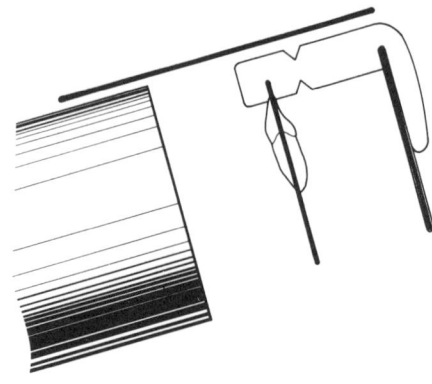

Horizontal angulation ►

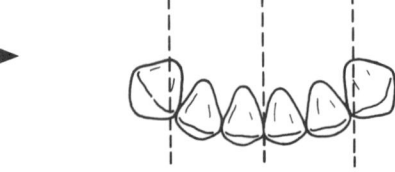

◄ **Centering**

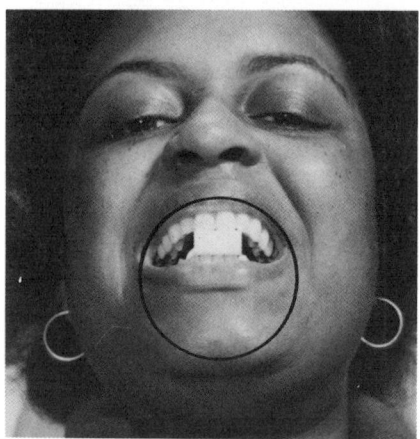

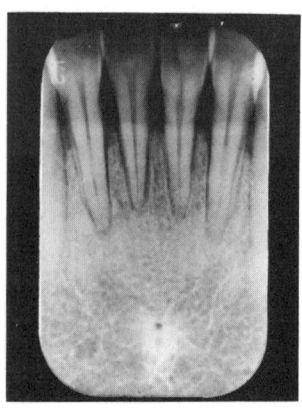

Fig. 21, V-5 Mandibular central incisors projection. Central and lateral incisors are shown. (Adapted from *Intraoral Radiography: The Paralleling Technique,* by Cy Whaley [Chapel Hill, N.C.: University of North Carolina, 1977])

STABE PARALLELING TECHNIQUE
Mandibular Lateral Incisor—Canine

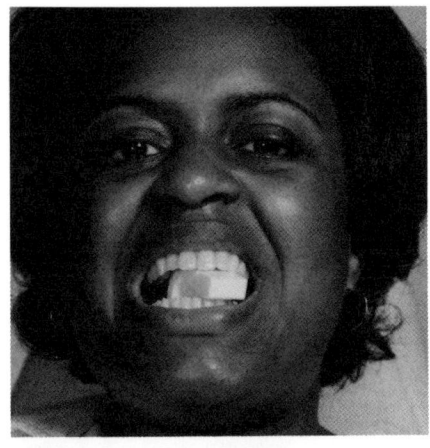

◄ **Packet placement** ►

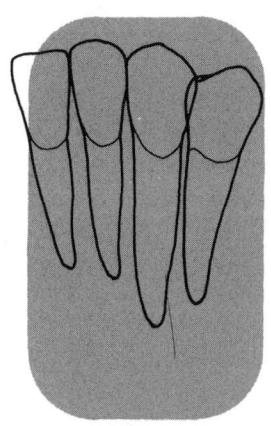

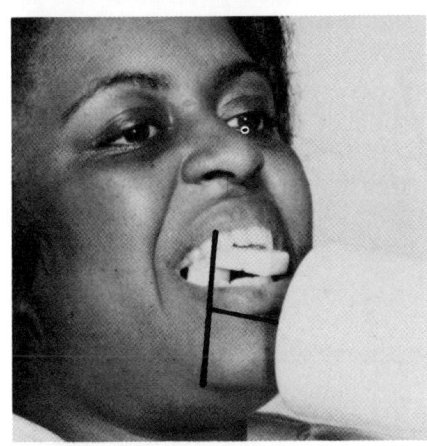

◄ **Vertical angulation** ►

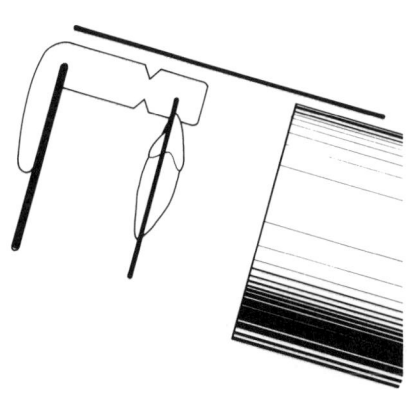

Horizontal angulation ►

◄ **Centering**

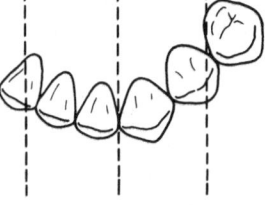

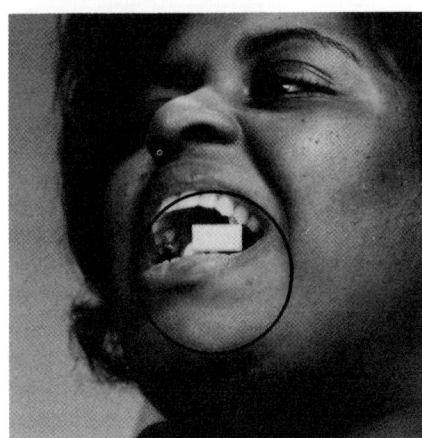

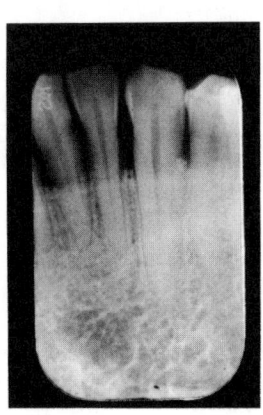

Fig. 22, V-5 Mandibular lateral incisor-canine projection. Lateral incisor and canine are shown. (Adapted from *Intraoral Radiography: The Paralleling Technique*, by Cy Whaley [Chapel Hill, N.C.: University of North Carolina, 1977])

STABE PARALLELING TECHNIQUE
Mandibular Premolar

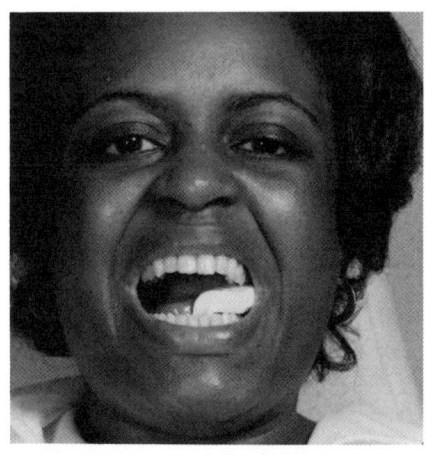

◄ **Packet placement** ►

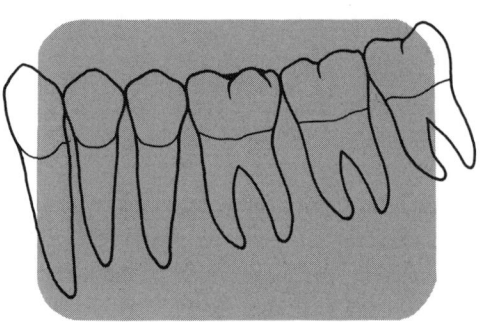

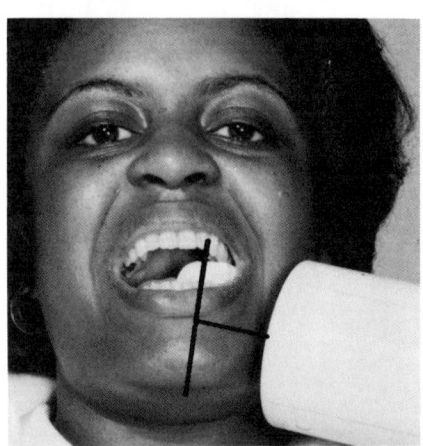

◄ **Vertical angulation** ►

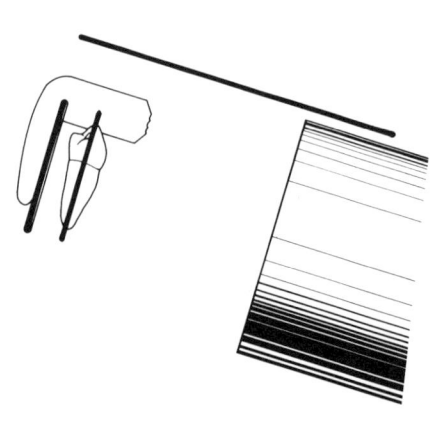

Horizontal angulation ►

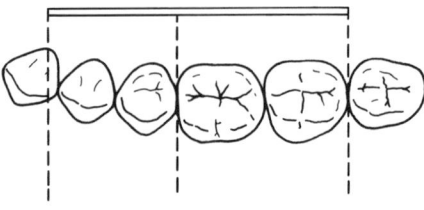

◄ **Centering**

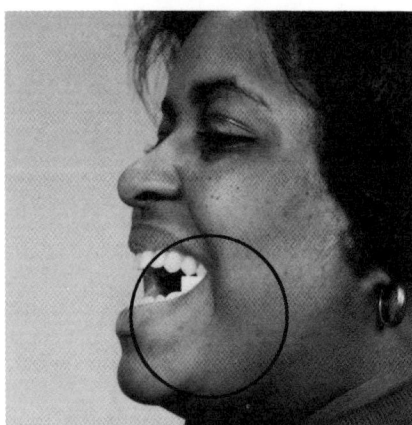

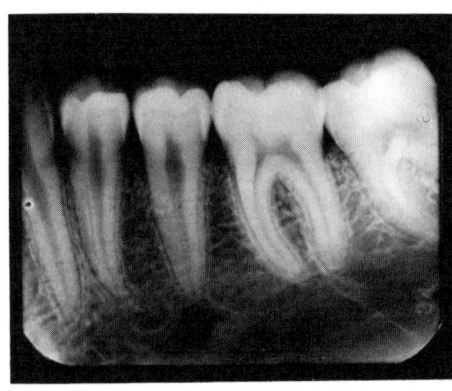

Fig. 23, V-5 Mandibular premolar projection. Distal half of canine, both premolars and first molar are shown. (Adapted from *Intraoral Radiography: The Paralleling Technique*, by Cy Whaley [Chapel Hill, N.C.: University of North Carolina, 1977])

STABE PARALLELING TECHNIQUE
Mandibular Molar

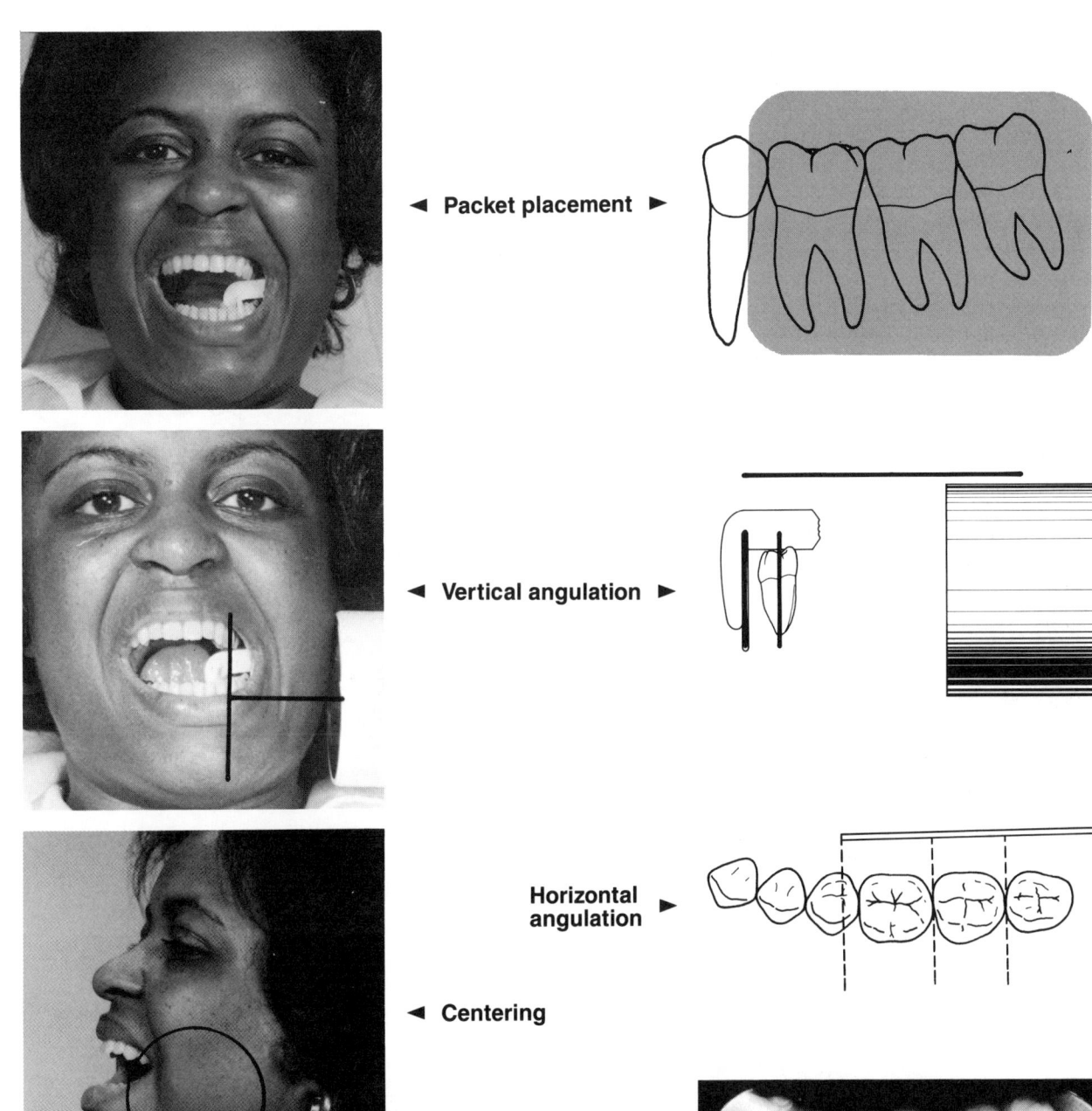

◄ **Packet placement** ►

◄ **Vertical angulation** ►

Horizontal angulation ►

◄ **Centering**

Fig. 24, V-5 Mandibular molar projection. First, second, and third molars are shown. (Adapted from *Intraoral Radiography: The Paralleling Technique*, by Cy Whaley [Chapel Hill, N.C.: University of North Carolina, 1977])

Bitewing Technique

The bitewing radiograph demonstrates the crowns of the maxillary and mandibular teeth and the crests of the alveolar ridges. A bite tab is manufactured or added to the packet to ensure correct placement for recording the maxillary crowns along the top half and the mandibular crowns along the bottom half of the film. The diagnosis of interproximal caries and evaluation of the crest of the alveolar ridges is made from bitewing film. For most children under the age of 16, one premolar bitewing on each side is adequate to demonstrate the interproximal spaces of the posterior teeth. For adults, two bitewings on each side are usually required to demonstrate the interproximal spaces from the canine to the third molar. The patient's occlusal plane in the closed position should be parallel to the floor during the exposure of all bitewing films.

PREMOLAR BITEWING. The packet is placed with the mesial edge of the film located at least as far forward as the center of the mandibular canine. It is positioned with the patient biting on the tab so that the upper and lower halves of the film are symmetrically located beside the upper and lower teeth. The vertical angulation is set at +10 degrees, or aiming downward. The horizontal angulation is established by directing the beam through the second premolar and first molar interproximal space. The cone is then adjusted so as not to cone-cut the film (Fig. 25, V-5).

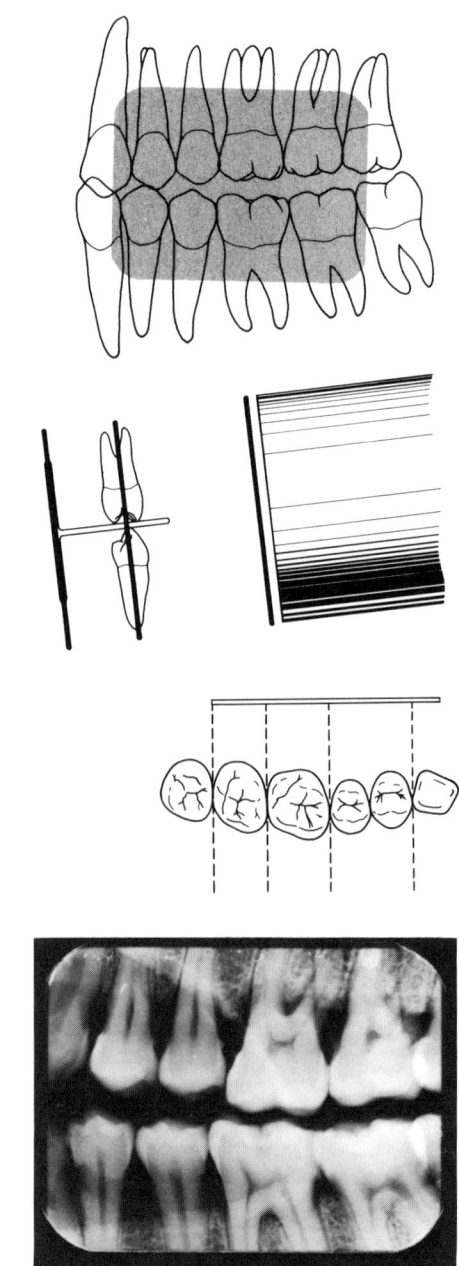

Fig. 25, V-5 Premolar bitewing projection. Shows interproximal spaces from canine to first molar.

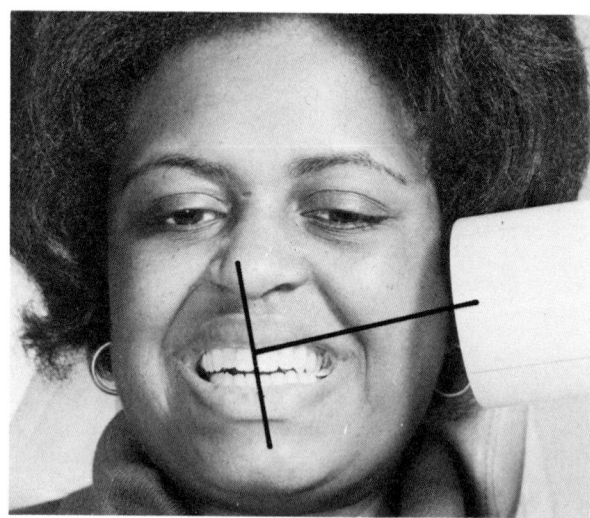

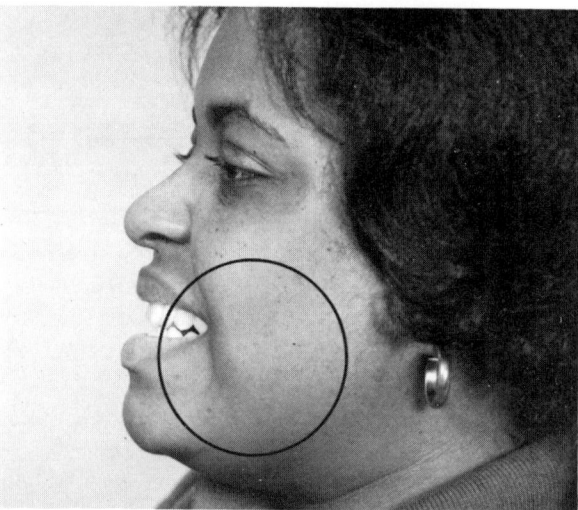

MOLAR BITEWING. The molar bitewing is needed for many patients in order to visualize properly the interproximal spaces between the molar teeth. The packet is placed with the mesial edge of the packet no farther forward than the center of the mandibular second premolar. The vertical angulation is +10 degrees and the horizontal angulation is established to open the interproximal spaces between the molar teeth (Fig. 26, V-5).

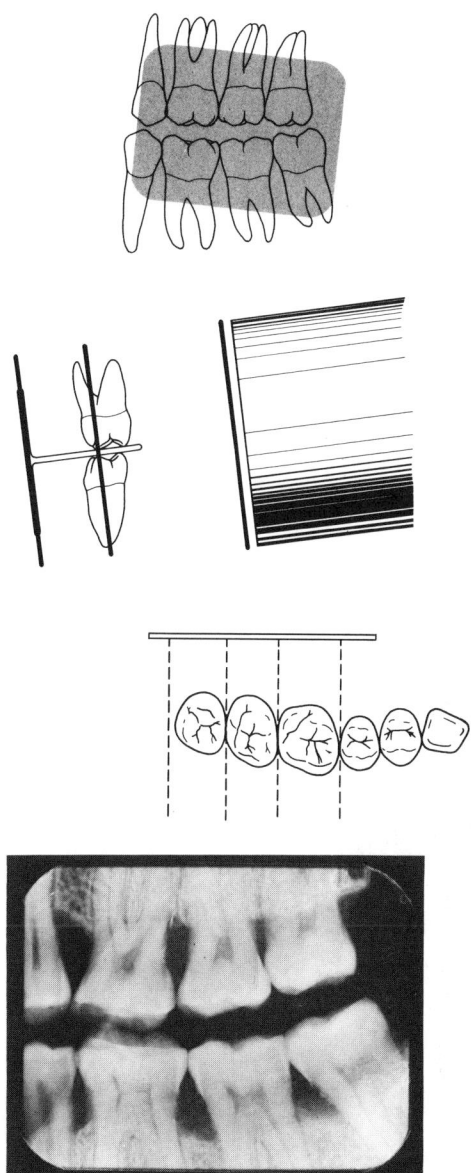

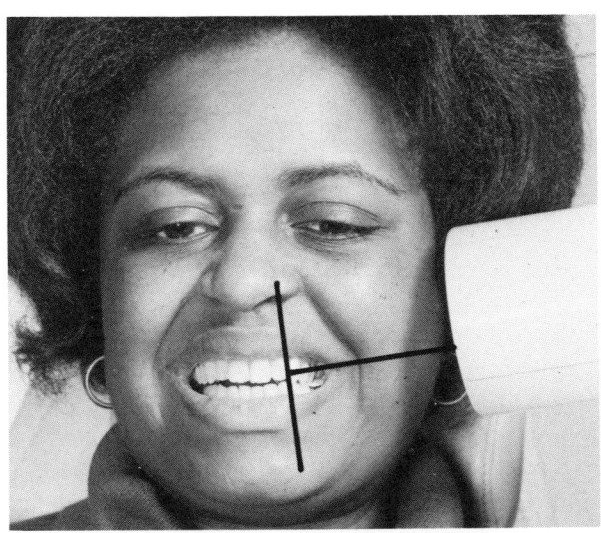

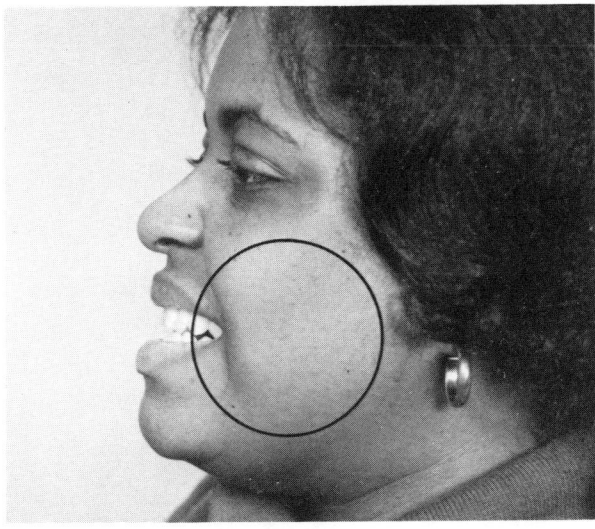

Fig. 26, V-5 Molar bitewing projection. Shows interproximal spaces of molars.

PRECISION INSTRUMENT PARALLELING TECHNIQUE

Lately, the Precision Instrument (Isaac Masel, Philadelphia, PA) has become available for use as a periapical film holder. These instruments consist of stainless steel components: cone-positioning disc, connecting bar, and a film holder. The components are constructed to align the x-ray beam and film in a parallel relationship that is consistent with the paralleling periapical technique. Precision Instruments are made in sizes for both adults and children, and an endodontic set is available. A major advantage of using these instruments is that the size of the x-ray beam is collimated by the opening in the center of the cone-positioning disc. The use of these instruments facilitates clinical periapical radiography and reduces x-ray exposure of the patient by about 60 percent. The clinical use of Precision Instruments for an adult is illustrated in Figures 27–36, V-5.

PRECISION INSTRUMENT PARALLELING TECHNIQUE
Maxillary Central Incisor

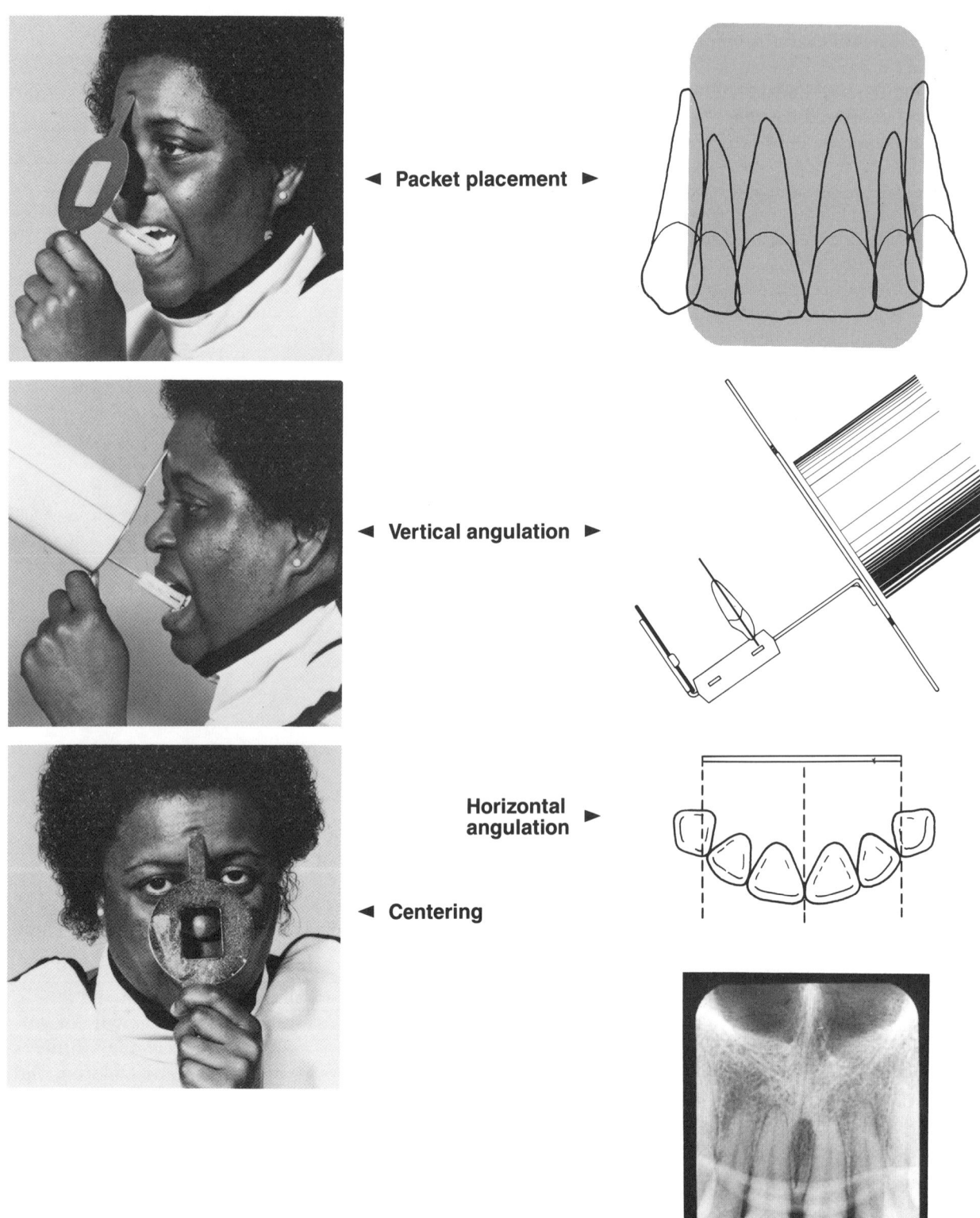

◄ **Packet placement** ►

◄ **Vertical angulation** ►

Horizontal angulation ►

◄ **Centering**

Fig. 27, V-5 Maxillary central incisor projection. Central and lateral incisors are shown.

PRECISION INSTRUMENT PARALLELING TECHNIQUE
Maxillary Lateral Incisor—Canine

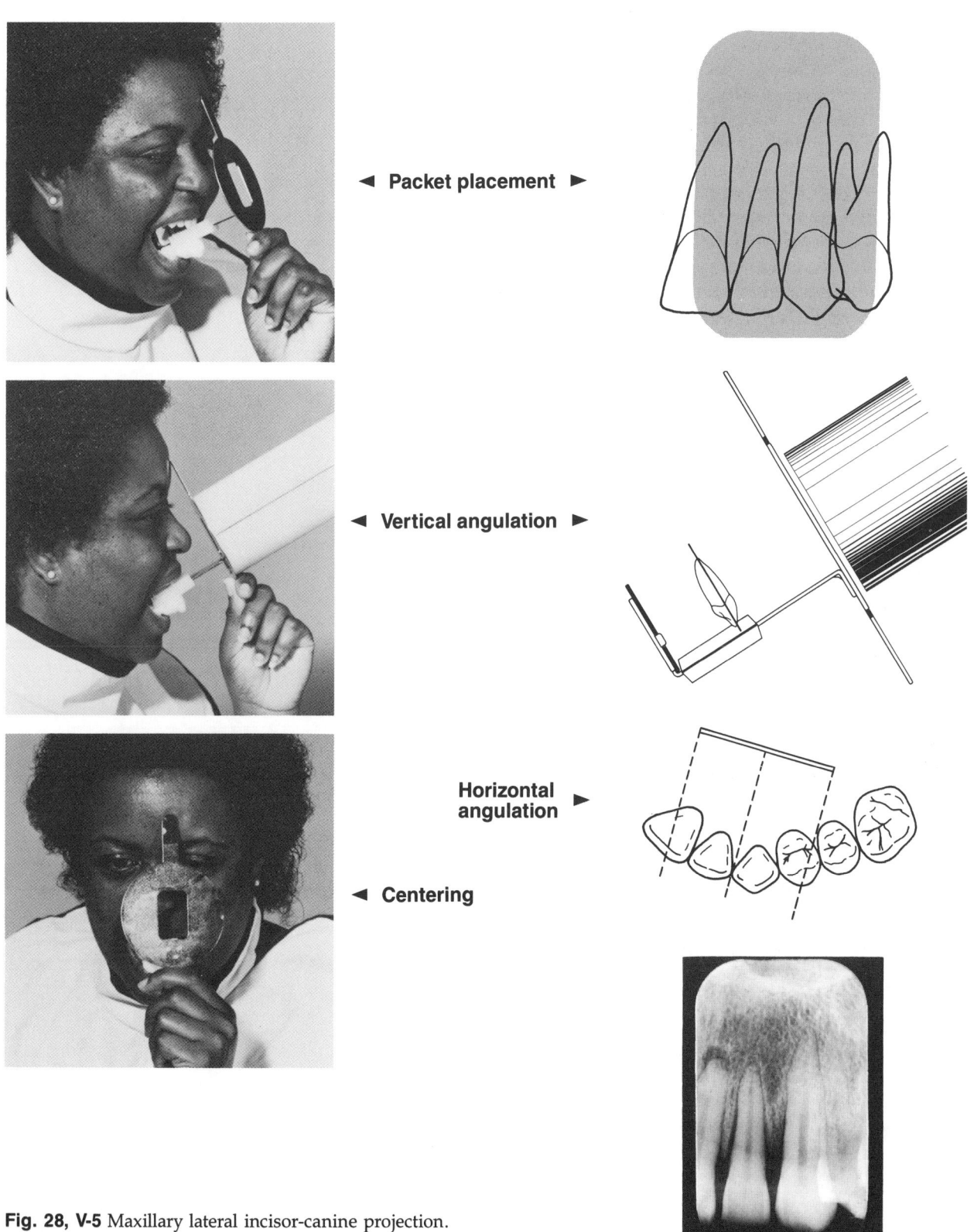

◄ **Packet placement** ►

◄ **Vertical angulation** ►

Horizontal angulation ►

◄ **Centering**

Fig. 28, V-5 Maxillary lateral incisor-canine projection.
Lateral incisor and canine are shown.

PRECISION INSTRUMENT PARALLELING TECHNIQUE
Maxillary Premolar

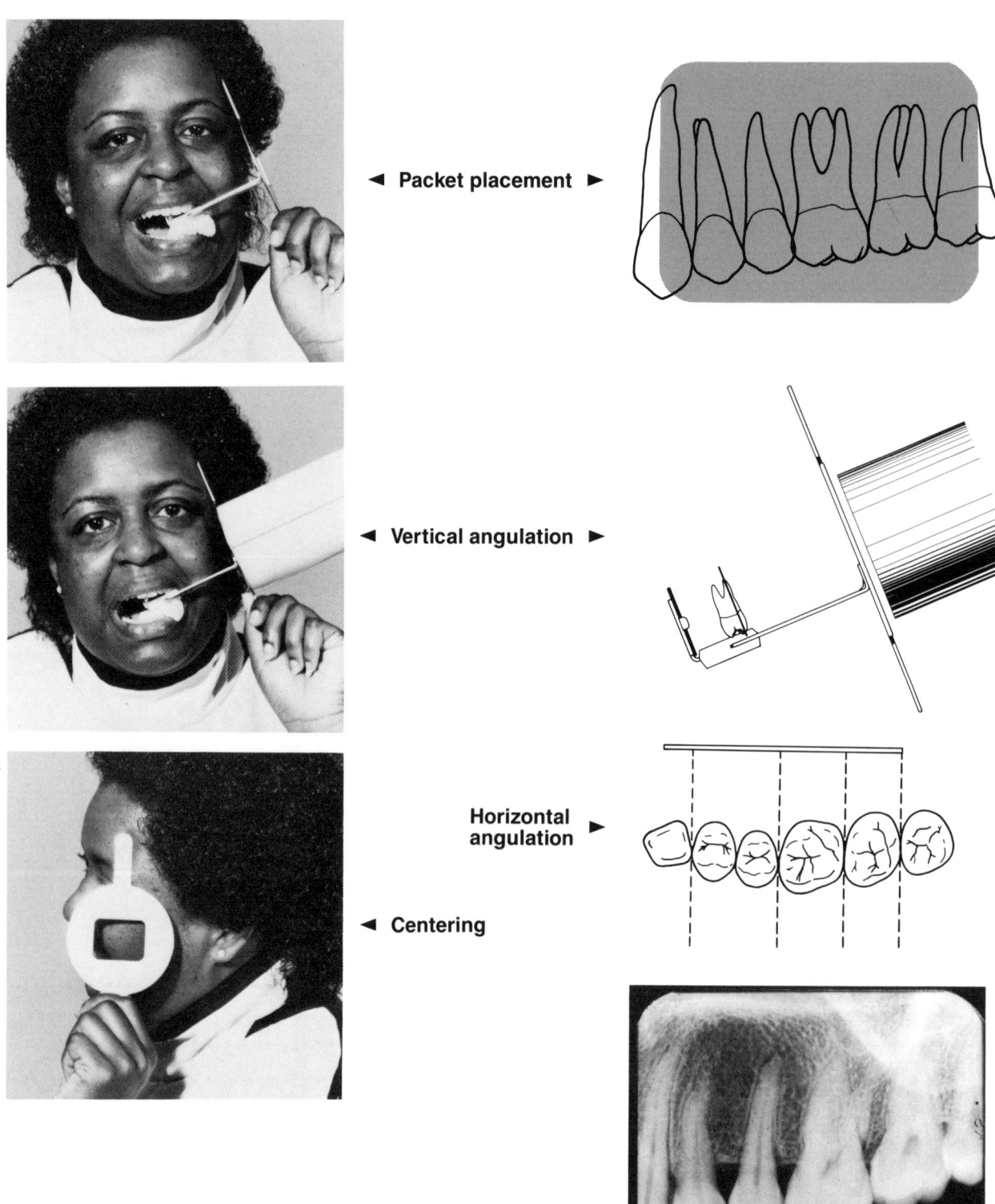

◄ **Packet placement** ►

◄ **Vertical angulation** ►

Horizontal angulation ►

◄ **Centering**

Fig. 29, V-5 Maxillary premolar projection. Distal half of canine, both premolars, and first molar are shown.

PRECISION INSTRUMENT PARALLELING TECHNIQUE
Maxillary Molar

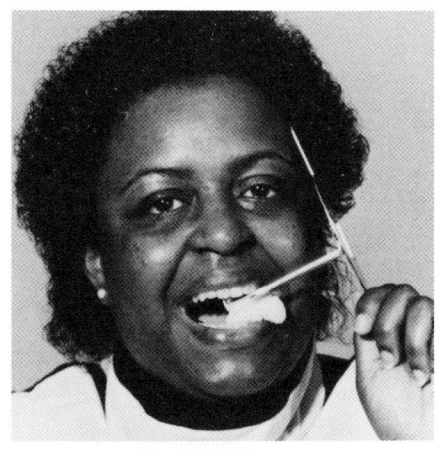

◄ **Packet placement** ►

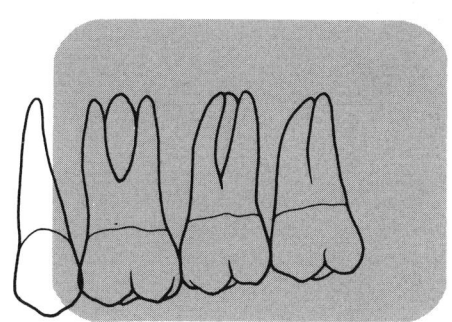

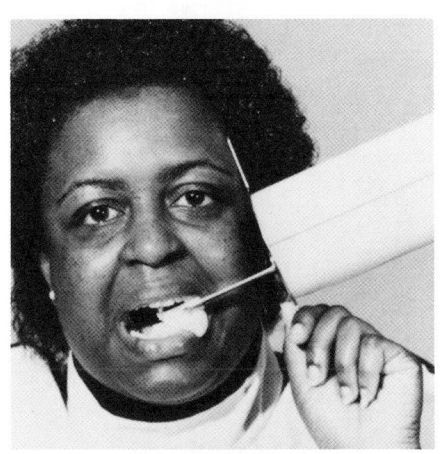

◄ **Vertical angulation** ►

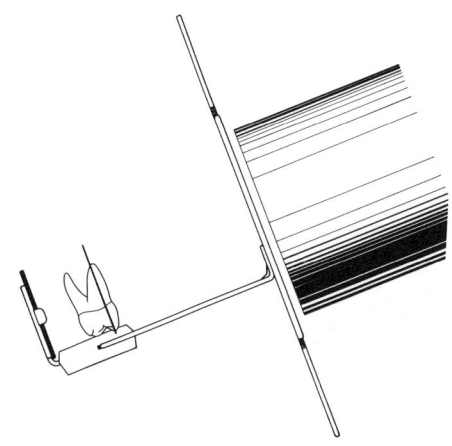

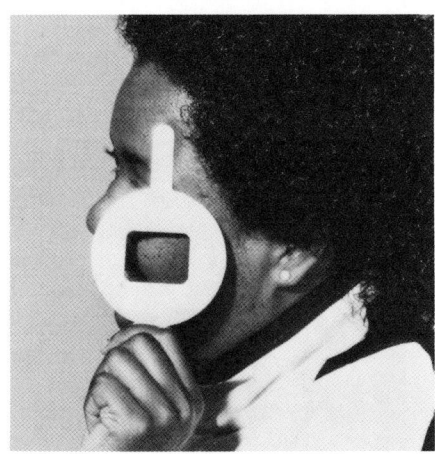

Horizontal angulation ►

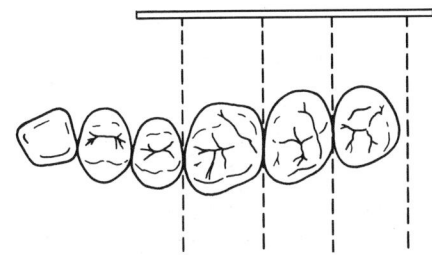

◄ **Centering**

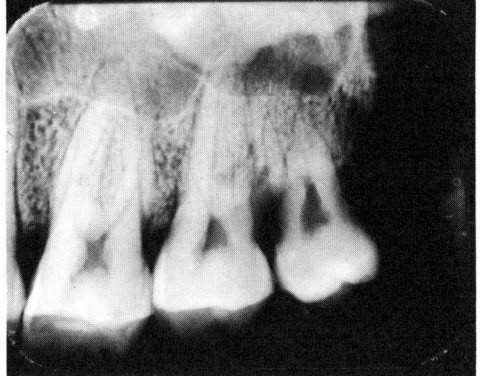

Fig. 30, V-5 Maxillary molar projection. First, second, and third molars are shown.

PRECISION INSTRUMENT PARALLELING TECHNIQUE
Mandibular Central Incisor

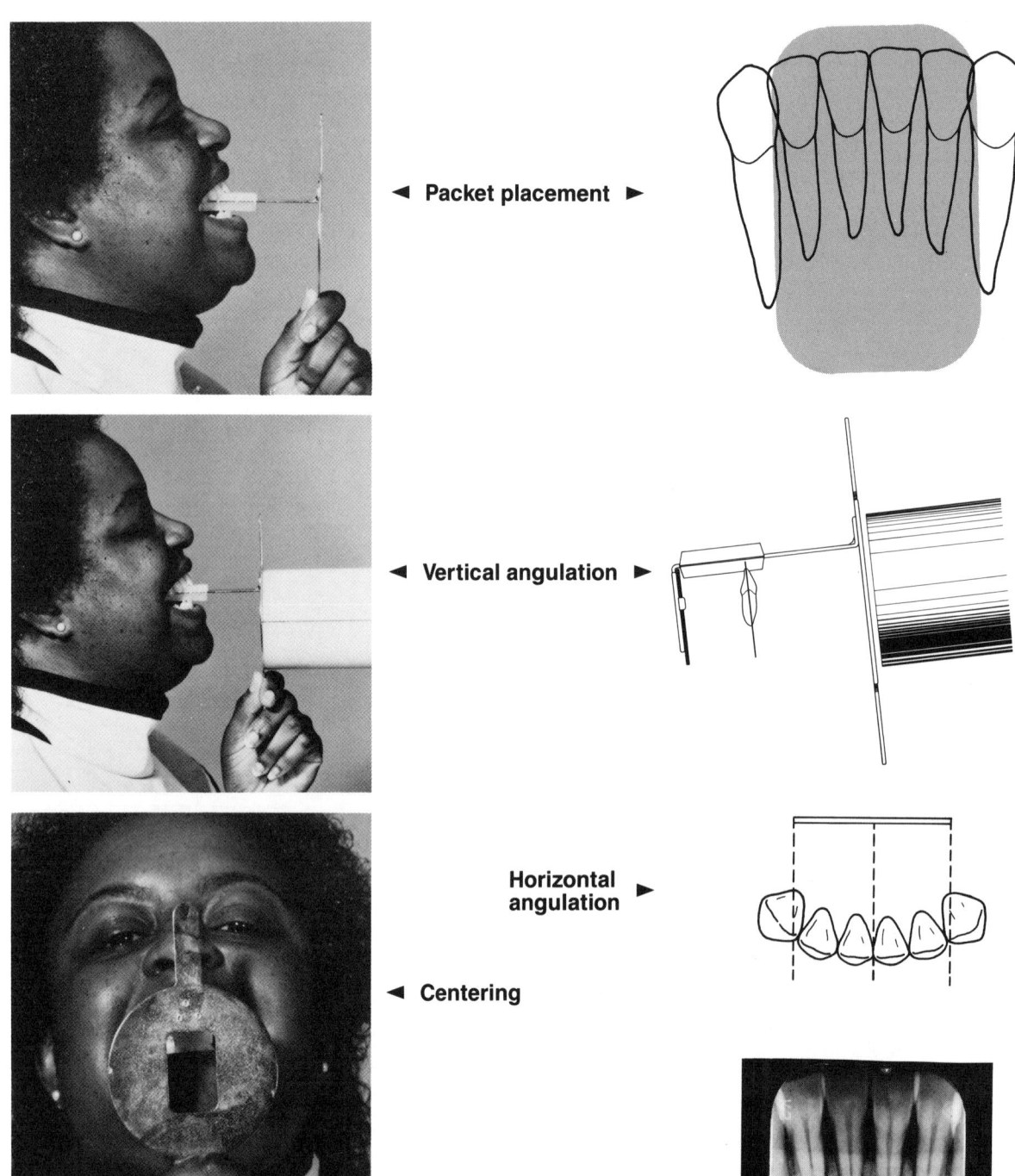

◄ **Packet placement** ►

◄ **Vertical angulation** ►

Horizontal angulation ►

◄ **Centering**

Fig. 31, V-5 Mandibular central incisor projection. Central and lateral incisors are shown.

PRECISION INSTRUMENT PARALLELING TECHNIQUE
Mandibular Lateral Incisor—Canine

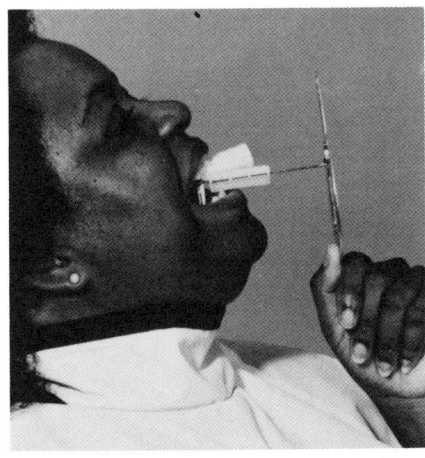

◄ **Packet placement** ►

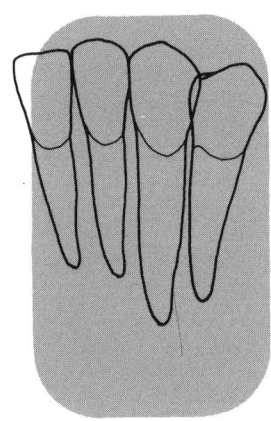

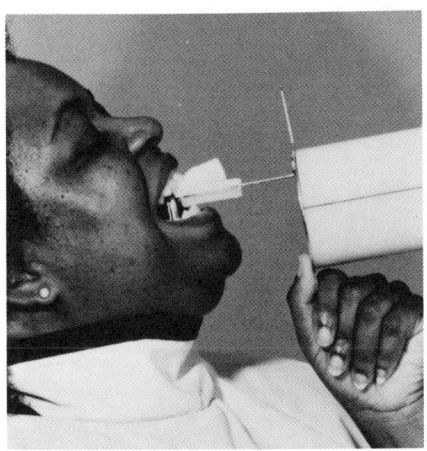

◄ **Vertical angulation** ►

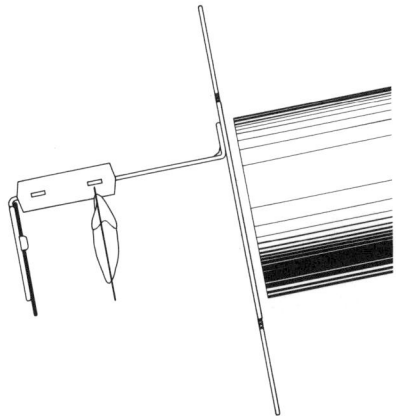

Horizontal angulation ►

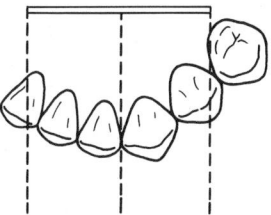

◄ **Centering**

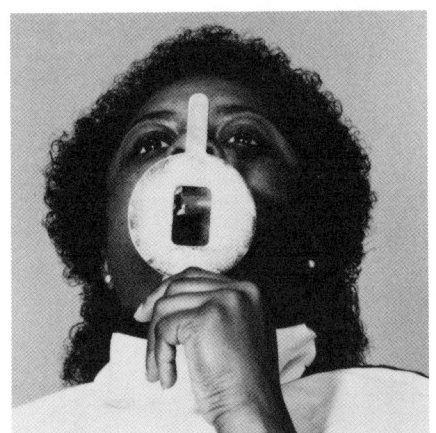
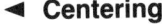

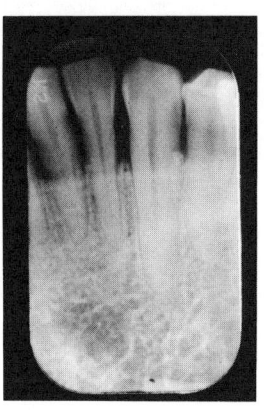

Fig. 32, V-5 Mandibular lateral incisor-canine projection. Lateral incisor and canine are shown.

PRECISION INSTRUMENT PARALLELING TECHNIQUE
Mandibular Premolar

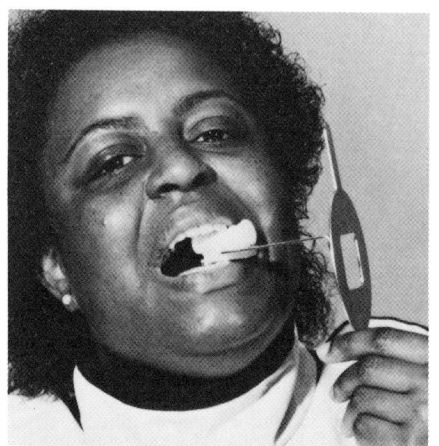

◄ **Packet placement** ►

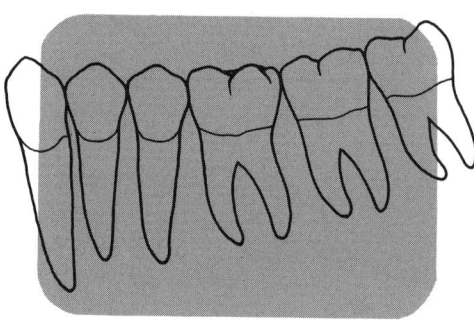

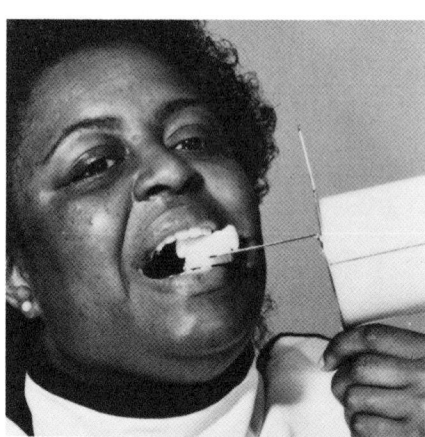

◄ **Vertical angulation** ►

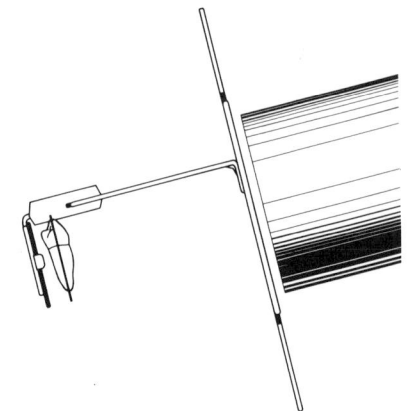

Horizontal angulation ►

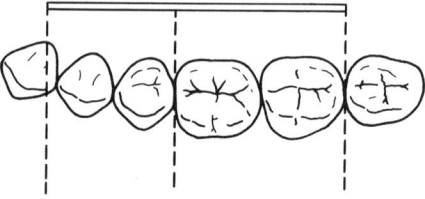

◄ **Centering**

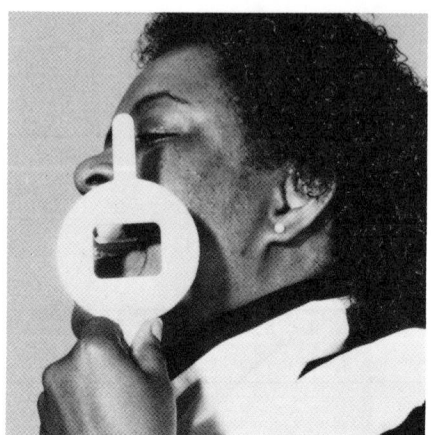

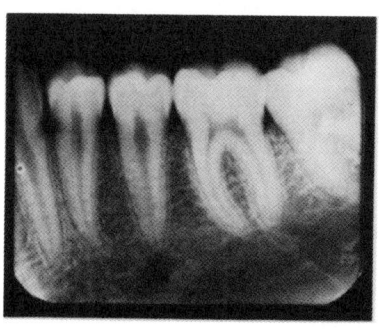

Fig. 33, V-5 Mandibular premolar projection. Distal one-half of canine, both premolars, and first molar are shown.

PRECISION INSTRUMENT PARALLELING TECHNIQUE
Mandibular Molar

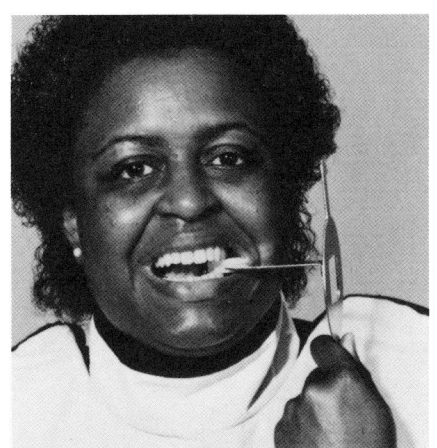

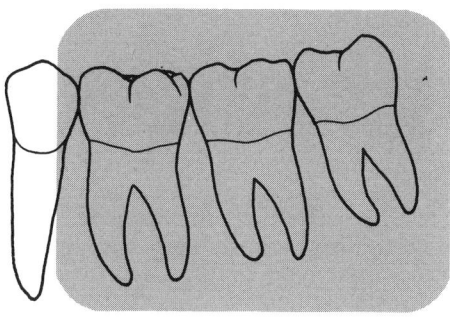

◄ **Packet placement** ►

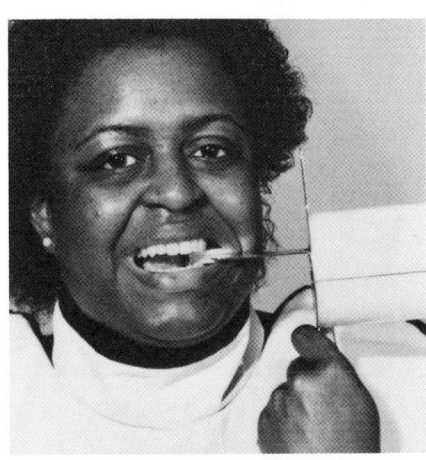

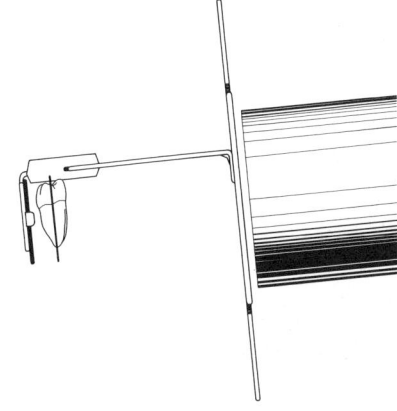

◄ **Vertical angulation** ►

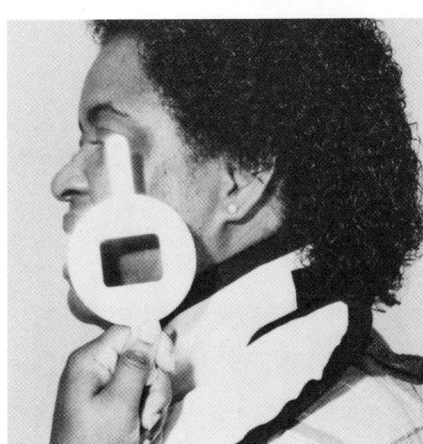

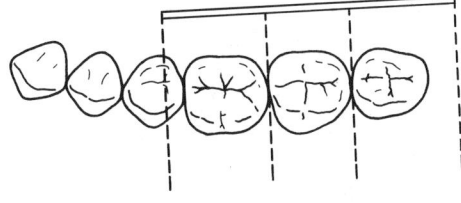

Horizontal angulation ►

◄ **Centering**

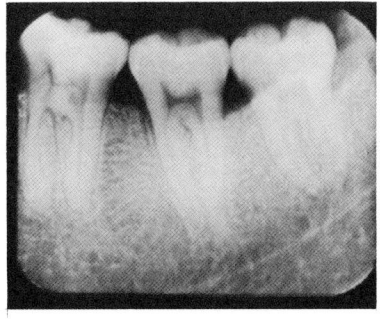

Fig. 34, V-5 Mandibular molar projection. First, second, and third molars are shown.

PRECISION INSTRUMENT BITEWING TECHNIQUE
Premolar Bitewing

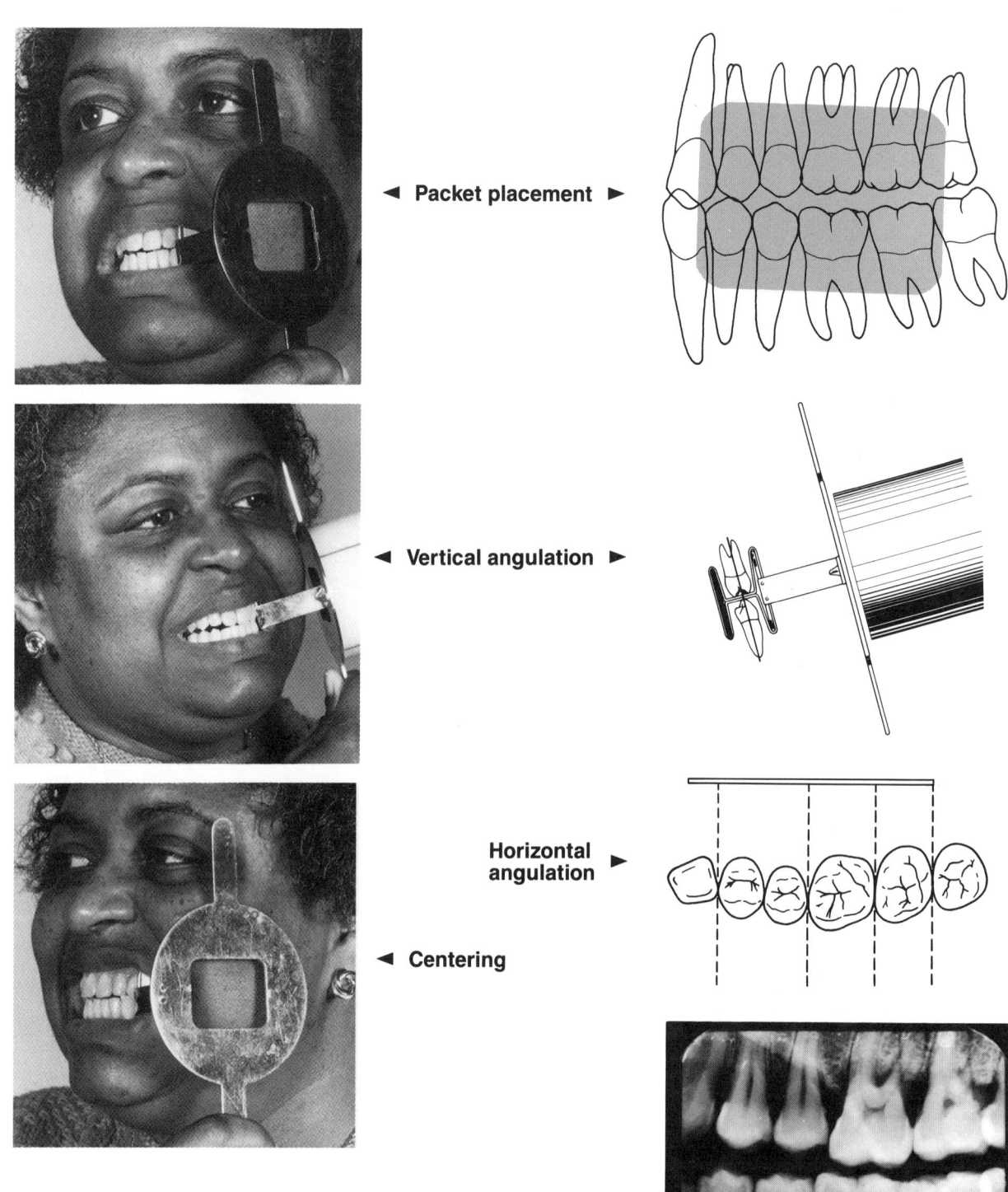

◄ **Packet placement** ►

◄ **Vertical angulation** ►

Horizontal angulation ►

◄ **Centering**

Fig. 35, V-5 Premolar bitewing projection. Shows interproximal spaces from canine to first molar.

PRECISION INSTRUMENT BITEWING TECHNIQUE
Molar Bitewing

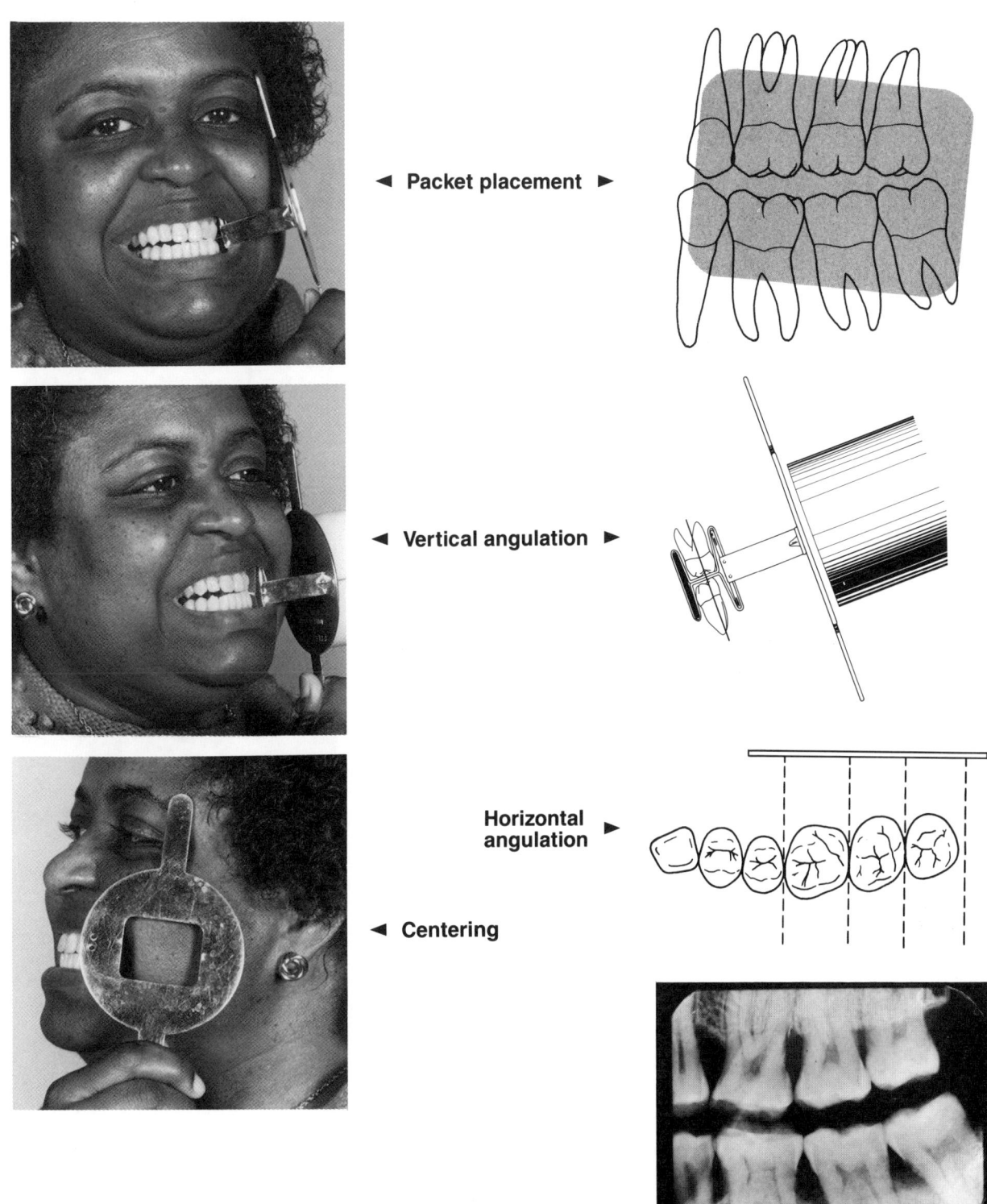

◄ **Packet placement** ►

◄ **Vertical angulation** ►

Horizontal angulation ►

◄ **Centering**

Fig. 36, V-5 Molar bitewing projection. Shows interproximal spaces of molars.

BISECTING-THE-ANGLE TECHNIQUE

Early in the twentieth century, the bisecting-the-angle technique was introduced by Cieszynski as the first standardized technique for obtaining periapical radiographs. The procedure was based on establishing the vertical angulation by applying the rule of isometry to dental radiography. The rule states that, if the angle formed by the plane of the film and the plane of the teeth is bisected, and the x-ray beam is directed at a right angle to the bisector, the image of the tooth on the film will be of correct length. The central ray is also directed through the apex of the root apex (Fig. 37, V-5).

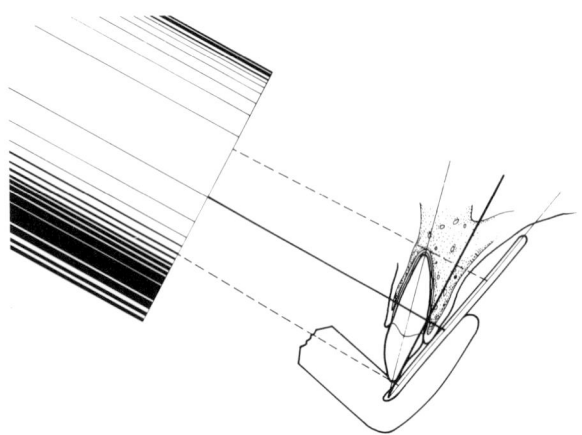

Fig. 37, V-5 Principle of the bisecting-the-angle method. X rays are directed perpendicular to the plane formed by the film and the long axis of the tooth.

PATIENT POSITION. Use of the bisecting-the-angle method requires careful positioning of the head of the patient. For both maxillary and mandibular projections the sagittal plane must be perpendicular to the floor. The occlusal plane of the arch being radiographed must be parallel to the floor (Figs. 38, 39, V5).

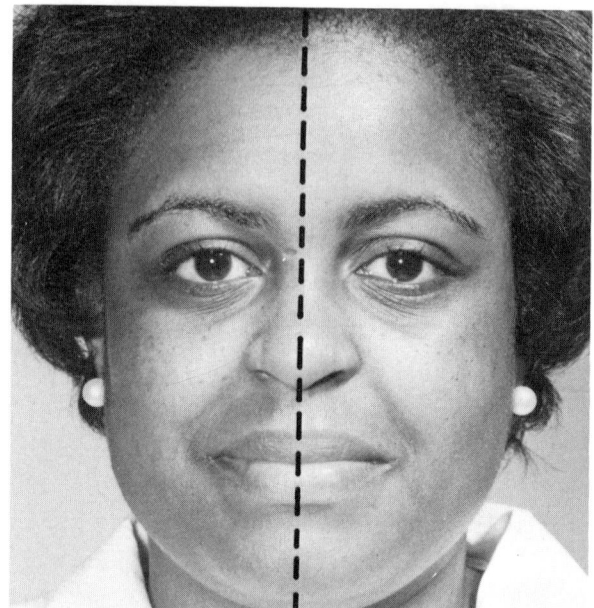

Fig. 38, V-5 Positioning patient for maxillary projections when using the bisecting-the-angle method.
    A. Mid-sagittal plane perpendicular to floor.

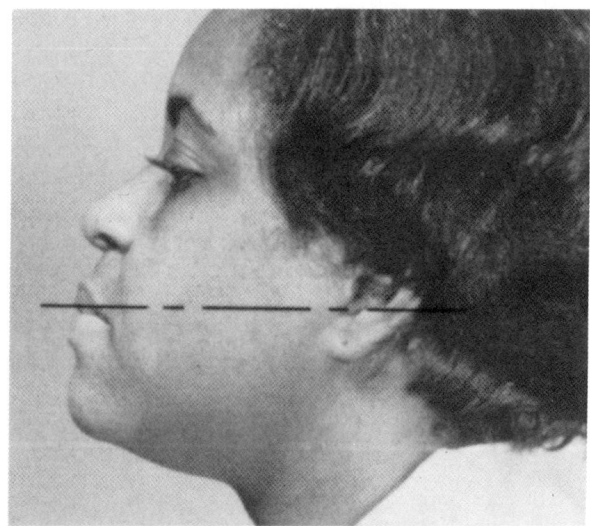

B. Maxillary occlusal plane parallel to floor.

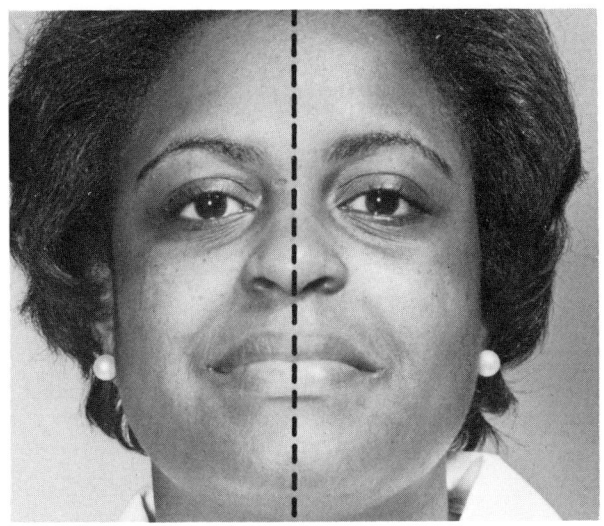

Fig. 39, V-5 Positioning the patient for mandibular projections when using the bisecting-the-angle method. A. Mid-sagittal plane perpendicular to floor.

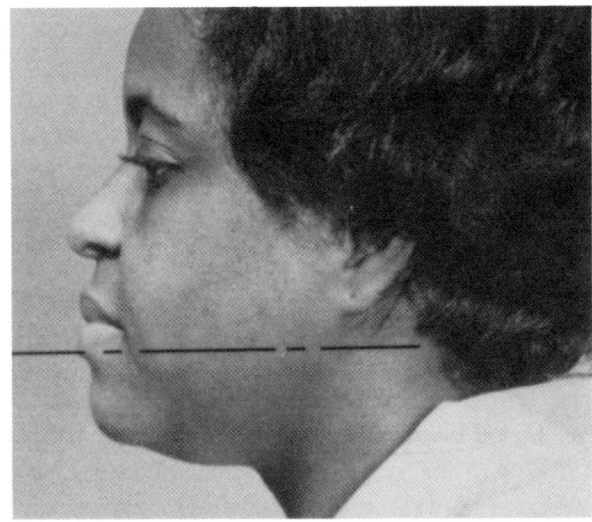

B. Mandibular occlusal plane parallel to floor.

Four Rules of Procedure for the Bisecting-the-Angle Technique

Rule 1. *Packet Placement: Place the film packet directly against the teeth and arch to be included in the projection.* The occlusal edge of the film should be even with the occlusal surfaces of the teeth. A film holder such as the Stabe or the Snap-a-ray is used to position the packet. The removable end of the Stabe is removed for placement of all periapical packets with this technique. The practice of having the patient stabilize the film packet with a finger has been discarded because of the unnecessary radiation exposure to the fingers. Figure 40, V-5 demonstrates correct packet placement for the bisecting-the-angle technique.

Rule 2. *Vertical Angulation: Align the central ray at a right angle to the imaginary line formed by bisecting-the-angle formed by the intersection of the tooth plane and the film plane.* Figure 41, V-5 illustrates the positioning of the cone so that the central ray is perpendicular to the bisector. This relationship of cone to film and tooth will result in the correct length of teeth images. Errors in vertical angulation result in incorrect reproduction of the length of the tooth. If the vertical angle is too steep or too high, a degree angle is registered on the dial on the side of the tubehead, the images of the teeth will be too short (foreshortened). If the vertical angle is set not steep enough or too low, a degree angle is registered on the dial, the tooth images will be elongated (Fig. 42, V-5).

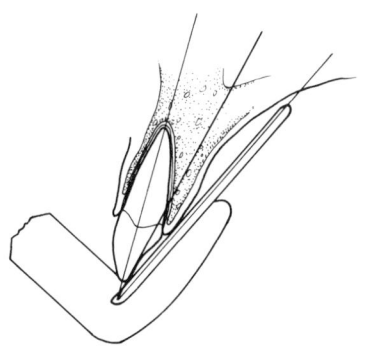

Fig. 40, V-5 Rule 1: Packet placement. Packet placed directly against teeth.

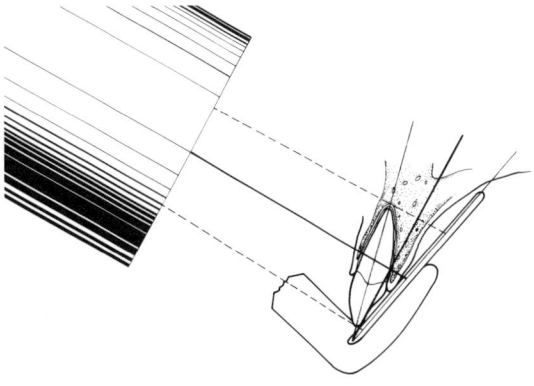

Fig. 41, V-5 Rule 2: Vertical angulation. X rays directed at a right angle to the imaginary bisector.

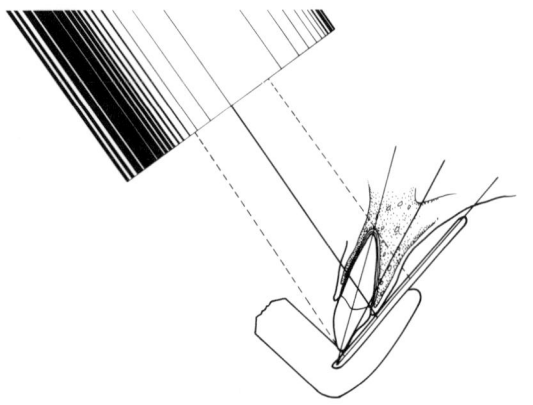

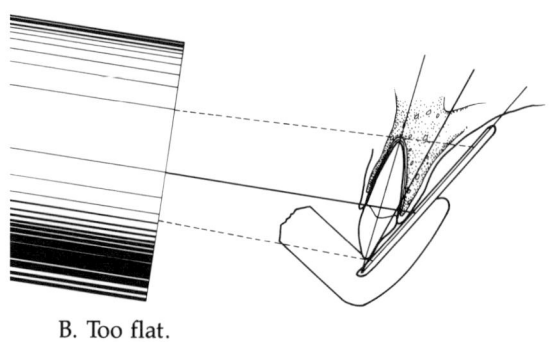

B. Too flat.

Fig. 42, V-5 Incorrect vertical angulation.
A. Too steep.

Rule 3. *Horizontal Angulation: Direct the x-ray beam through the spaces between the teeth.* Figure 43, V-5 demonstrates the principle of directing the x rays through the interproximal spaces, those spaces between the teeth. The diagnosis of caries is dependent on being able to see the mesial and distal surfaces of the teeth without overlapping of the adjacent tooth. After completing packet placement and vertical angulation, the operator should stand behind the tubehead and align the cone with the central ray through the interproximal surfaces of interest for the particular projection. Figure 44, V-5 illustrates incorrect horizontal alignment of the x-ray beam. Also shown is the appearance of overlapping interproximal spaces on both periapical and bitewing projections.

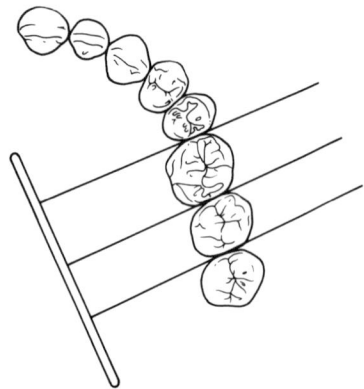

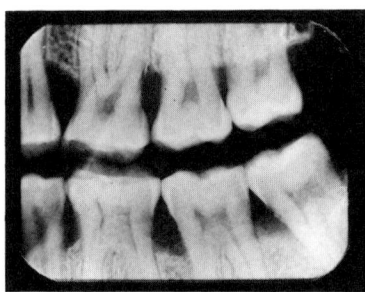

Fig. 43, V-5 Rule 3: Horizontal angulation.
A. Direct x rays through interproximal spaces.
B. Resulting radiograph.

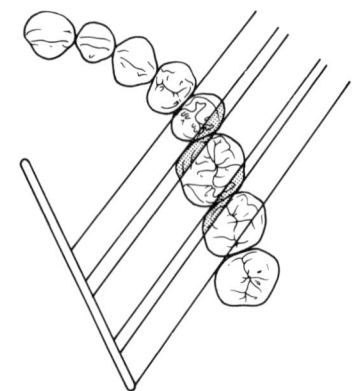

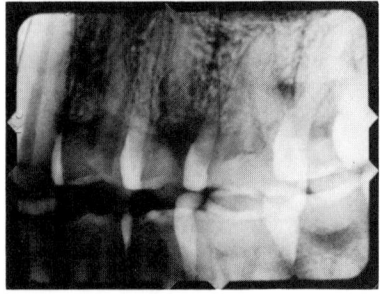

Fig. 44, V-5 Incorrect horizontal angulation.
A. Incorrect alignment of x-ray beam.
B. Resulting radiograph.

Rule 4. *Centering of the Exposure Field: Cover the film packet with the x-ray beam.* It is important that the x-ray beam cover the film packet. Failure to do this results in unexposed, clear areas on the film, called cone cuts. Even when the vertical and horizontal angulations are properly established, the cone can be out of position, causing some of the film to be missed by the x-ray beam. To prevent cone cuts, the cone should be aligned so that the open end of the cone is centered over the film packet. After establishing the vertical and horizontal angulations, minor changes in cone position are made by standing behind the tubehead and "sighting" down the sides of the cone. The operator should visualize that all four sides of the film packet will be exposed (Fig. 45, V-5). The broken-circle area demonstrates the correct cone position for a maxillary premolar projection, whereas the dark-circle area indicates the location of the cone during the exposure of the incorrect radiograph.

INDIVIDUAL PROJECTIONS. Figures 46-53, V-5 illustrate the packet placement, vertical and horizontal cone angulations, and centering of the exposure field for the eight standard projections using the bisecting-the-angle method. The Stabe holder is used with the end section removed, but the same principles apply when other film-holding devices are used.

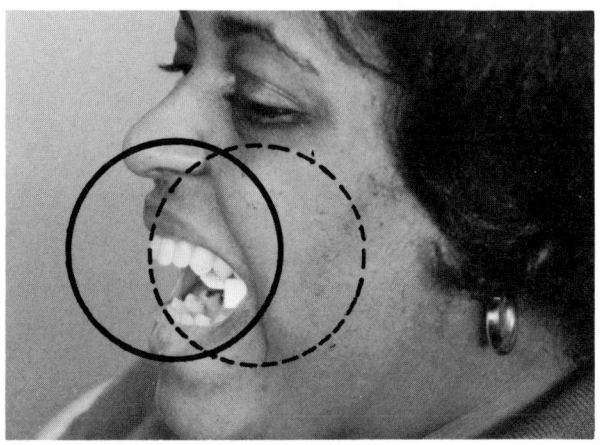

Fig. 45, V-5 Rule 4: Centering exposure field.
    A. Incorrect and correct centering of cone.

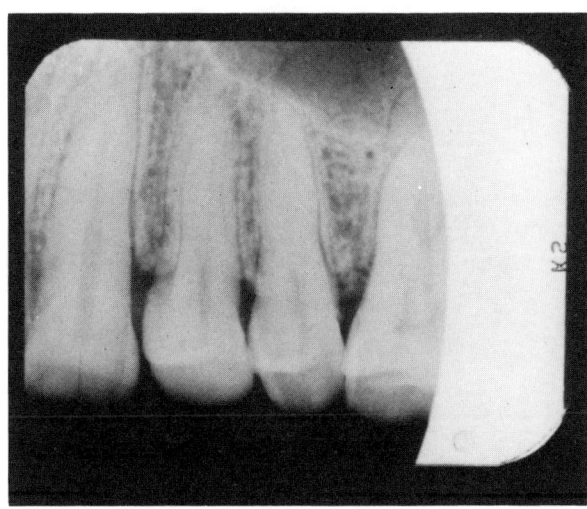

B. Resulting radiograph.

BISECTING-THE-ANGLE
Maxillary Central Incisor

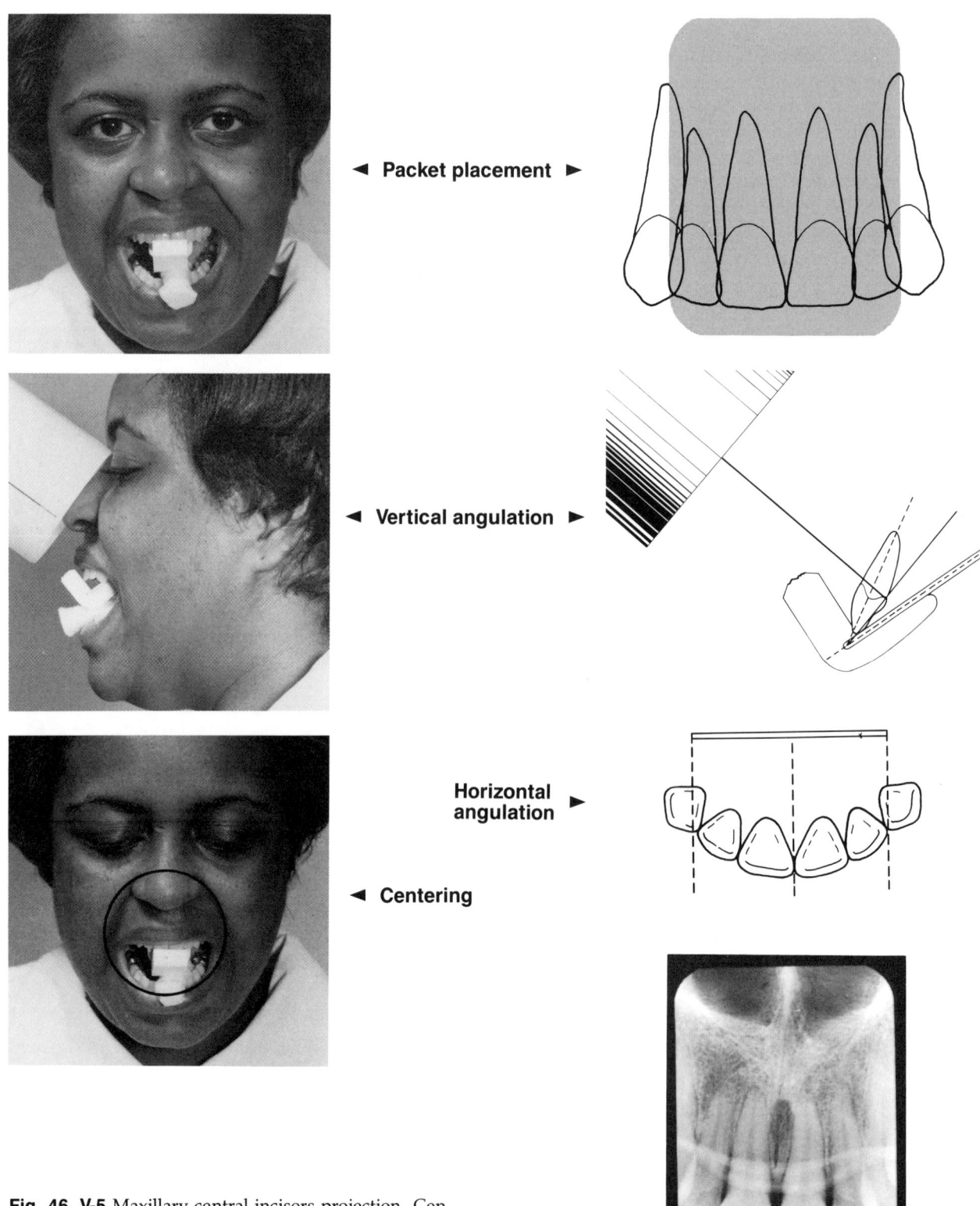

◄ **Packet placement** ►

◄ **Vertical angulation** ►

Horizontal angulation ►

◄ **Centering**

Fig. 46, V-5 Maxillary central incisors projection. Central and lateral incisors are shown. Vertical angulation is +55° to +65°.

BISECTING-THE-ANGLE
Maxillary Lateral Incisor—Canine

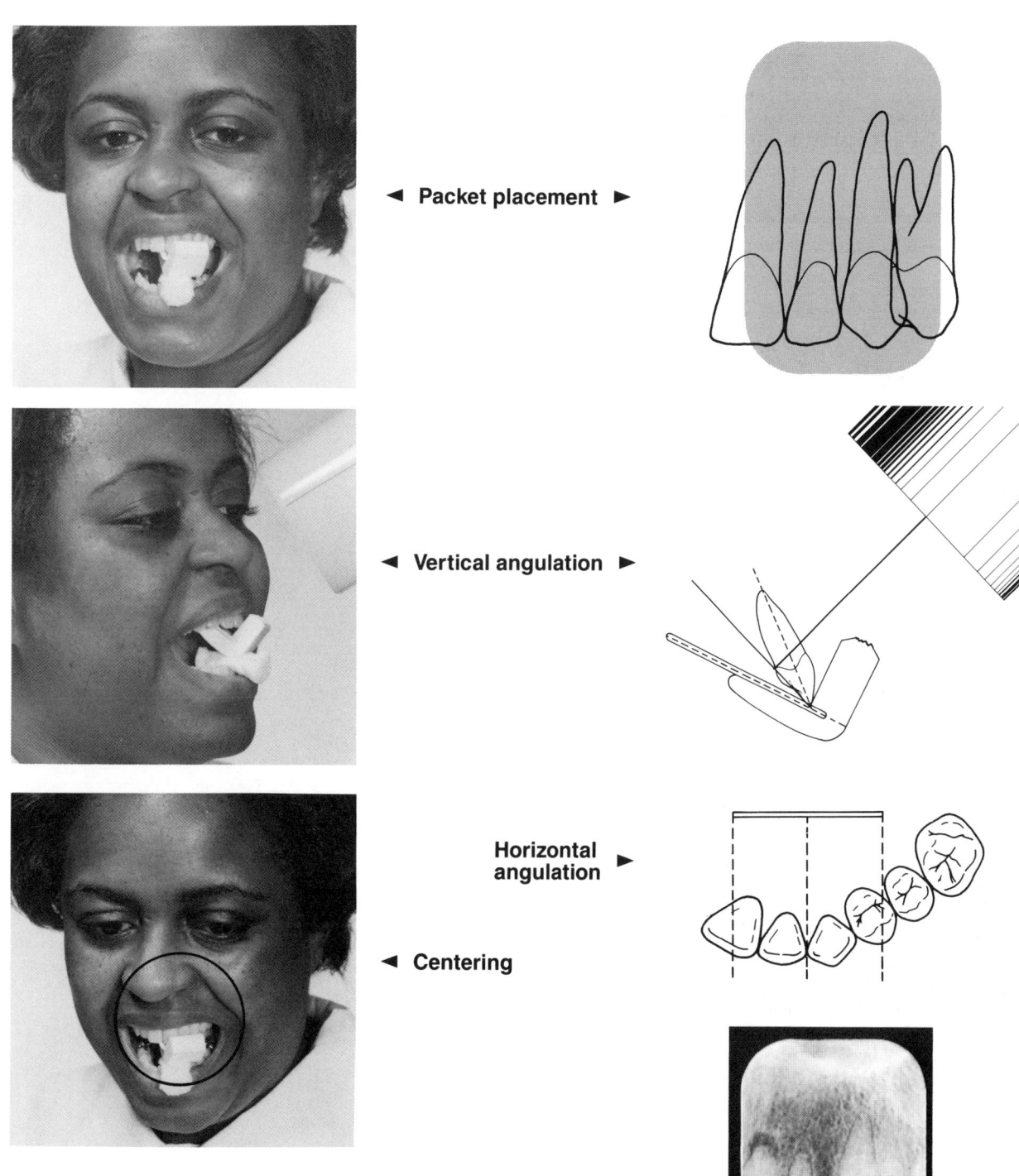

◄ **Packet placement** ►

◄ **Vertical angulation** ►

Horizontal angulation ►

◄ **Centering**

Fig. 47, V-5 Maxillary lateral incisor-canine projection. Lateral incisor and canine are shown. Vertical angulation is +45° to +50°.

BISECTING-THE-ANGLE
Maxillary Premolar

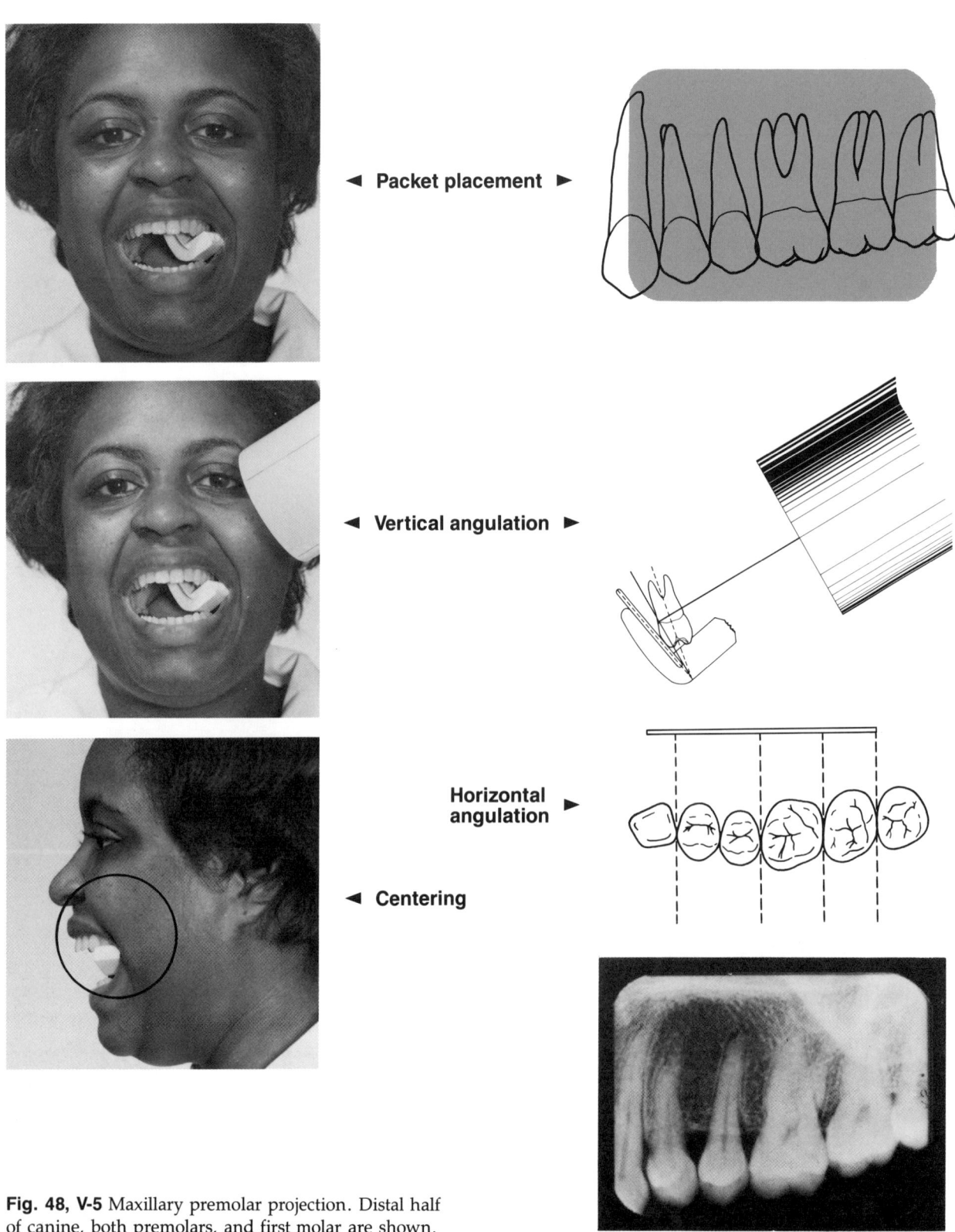

◄ **Packet placement** ►

◄ **Vertical angulation** ►

Horizontal angulation ►

◄ **Centering**

Fig. 48, V-5 Maxillary premolar projection. Distal half of canine, both premolars, and first molar are shown. Vertical angulation is +40°.

BISECTING-THE-ANGLE
Maxillary Molar

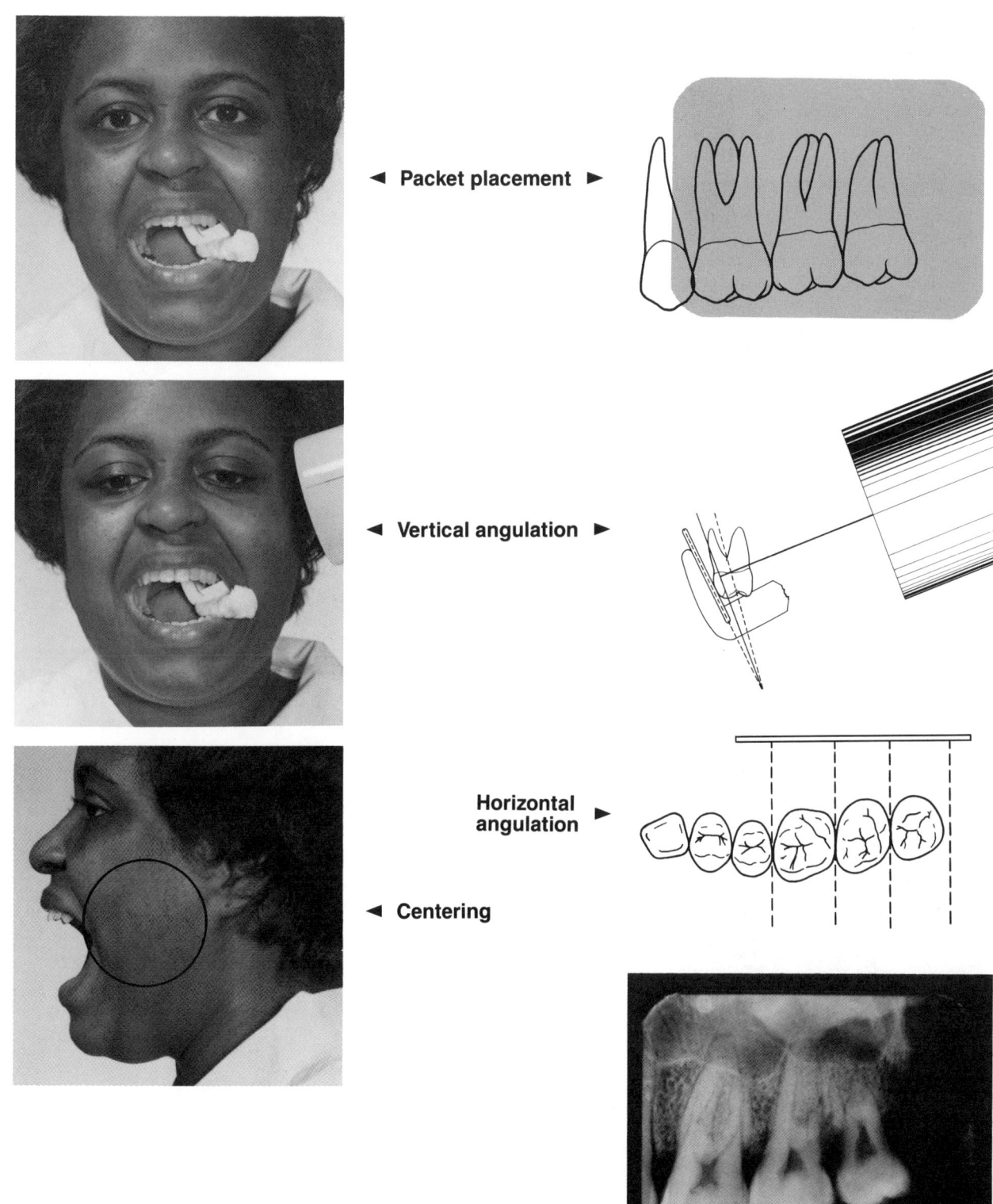

◄ **Packet placement** ►

◄ **Vertical angulation** ►

Horizontal angulation ►

◄ **Centering**

Fig. 49, V-5 Maxillary molar projection. First, second, and third molars are shown. Vertical angulation is +25° to +30°.

BISECTING-THE-ANGLE
Mandibular Central Incisor

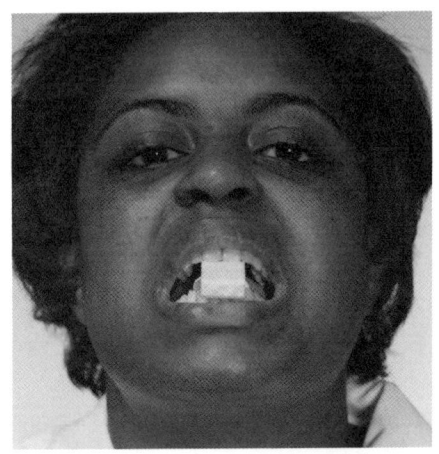

◄ **Packet placement** ►

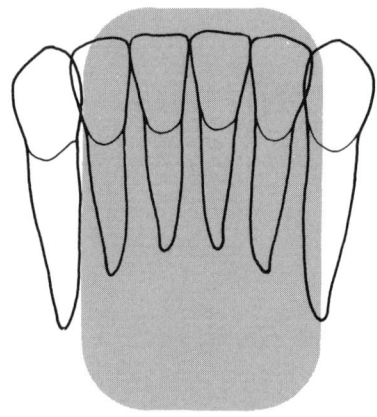

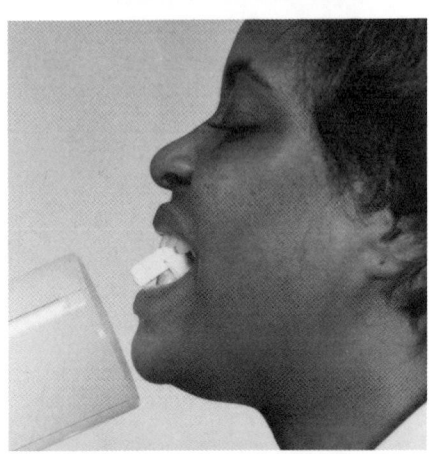

◄ **Vertical angulation** ►

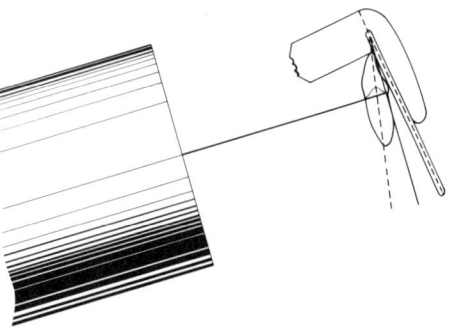

Horizontal angulation ►

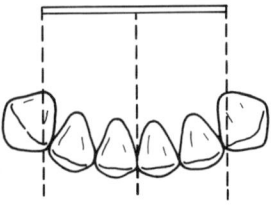

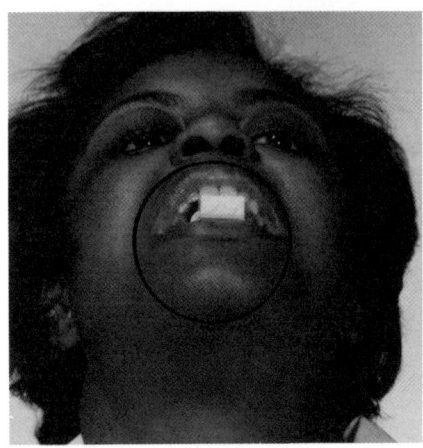

◄ **Centering**

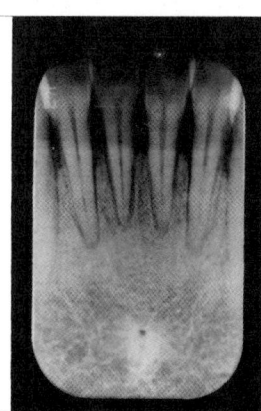

Fig. 50, V-5 Mandibular central incisors projection. Central incisors and lateral incisors are shown. Vertical angulation is −30°.

116

BISECTING-THE-ANGLE
Mandibular Lateral Incisor—Canine

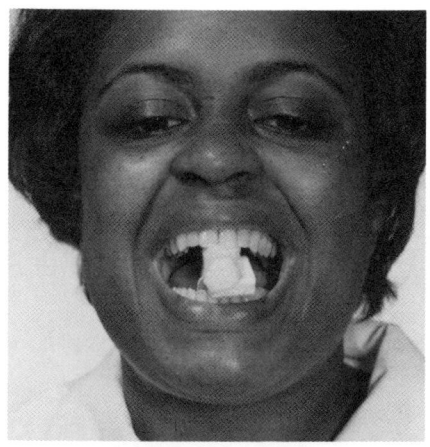

◄ **Packet placement** ►

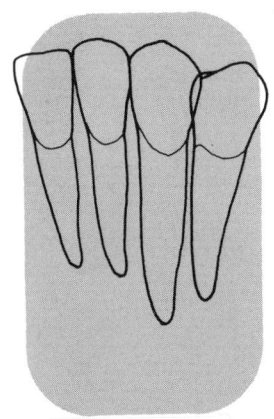

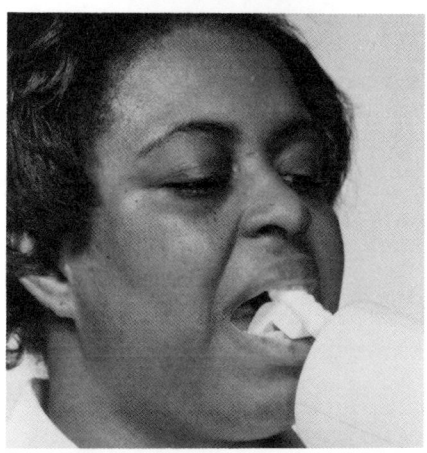

◄ **Vertical angulation** ►

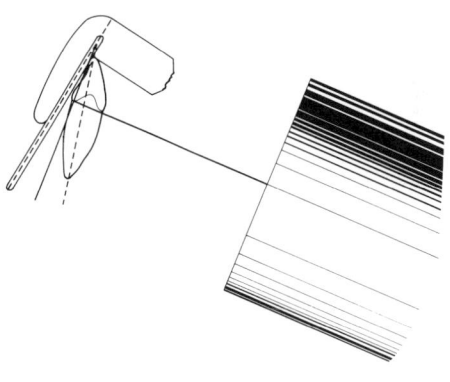

Horizontal angulation ►

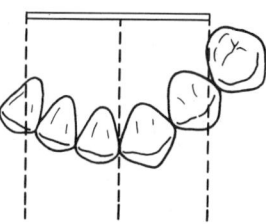

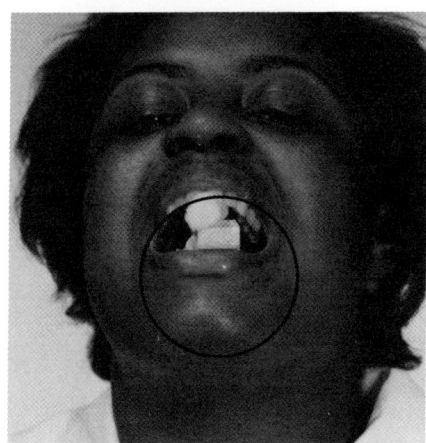

◄ **Centering**

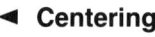

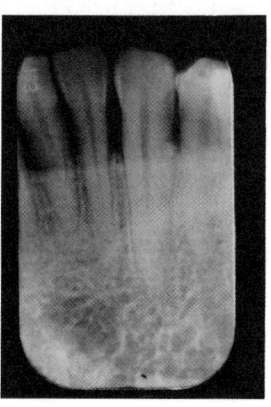

Fig. 51, V-5 Mandibular lateral incisor-canine projection. Lateral incisor and canine are shown. Vertical angulation is −30°.

BISECTING-THE-ANGLE
Mandibular Premolar

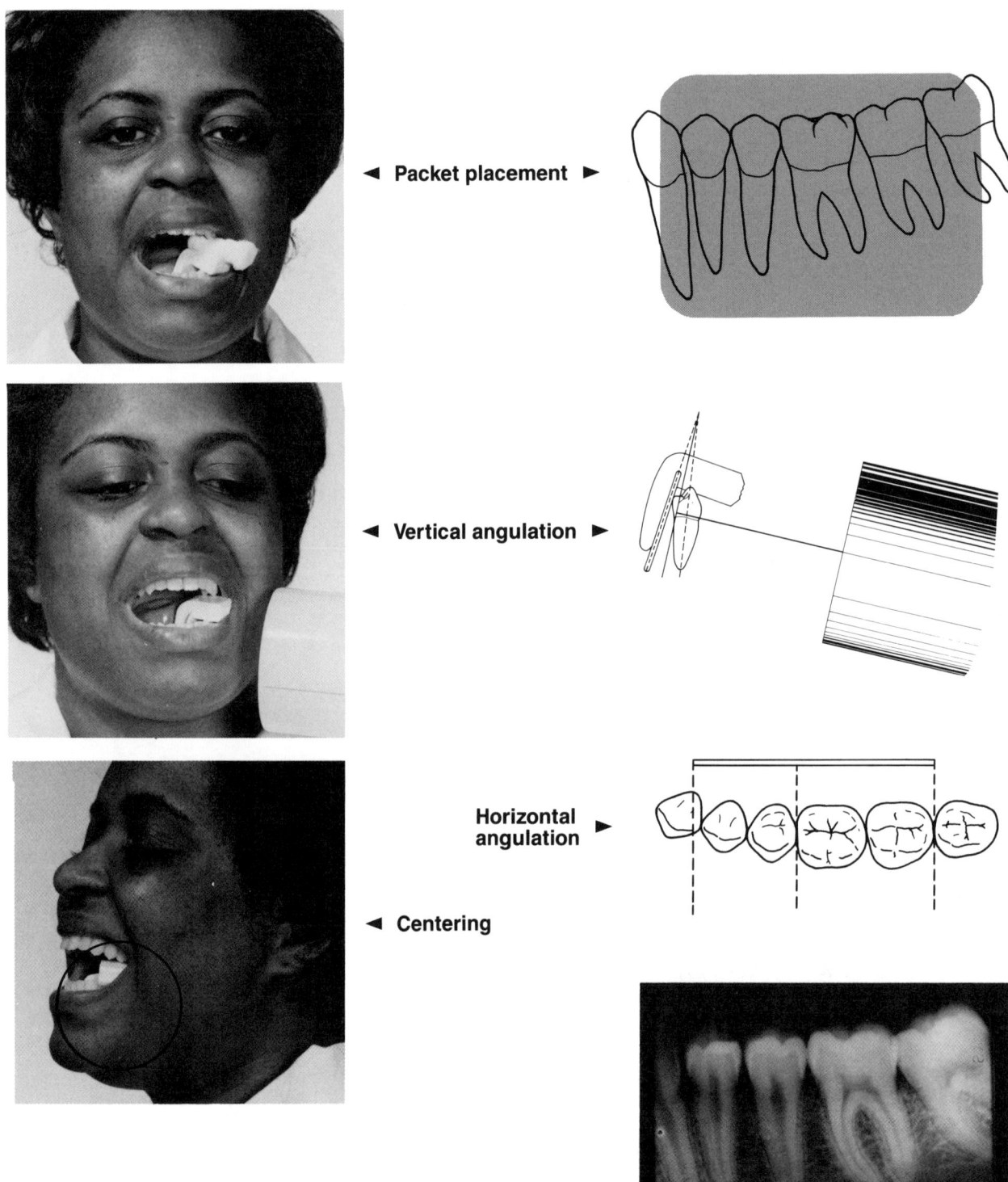

◄ **Packet placement** ►

◄ **Vertical angulation** ►

Horizontal angulation ►

◄ **Centering**

Fig. 52, V-5 Mandibular premolar projection. Distal half of canine, both premolars, and first molar are shown. Vertical angulation is −10°.

BISECTING-THE-ANGLE
Mandibular Molar

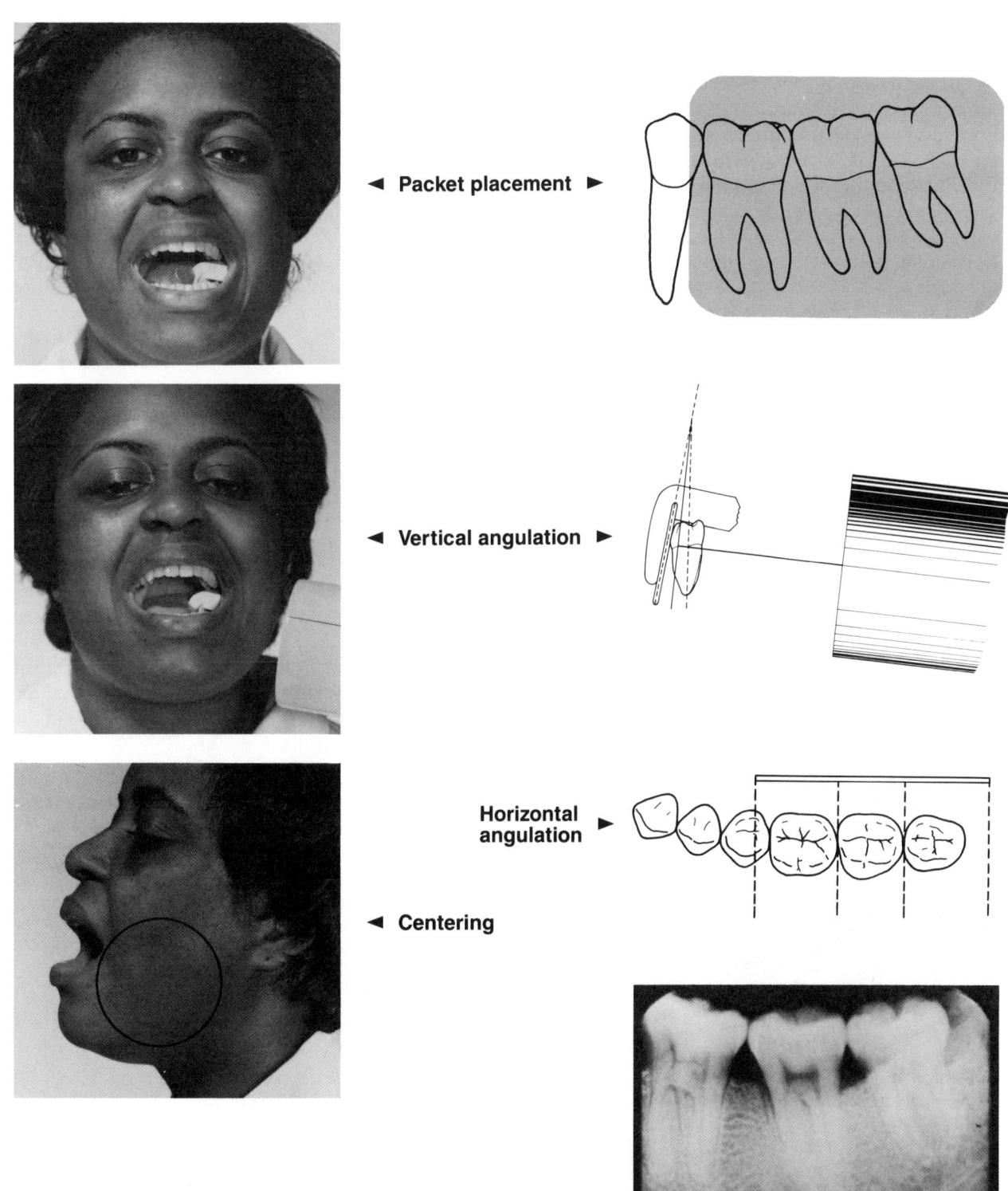

◄ **Packet placement** ►

◄ **Vertical angulation** ►

Horizontal angulation ►

◄ **Centering**

Fig. 53, V-5 Mandibular molar projection. First, second, and third molars are shown. Vertical angulation is 0°.

COMPARISON OF THE PARALLELING AND BISECTING-THE-ANGLE TECHNIQUES

An understanding of the advantages and disadvantages of the two commonly used periapical techniques enables the operator to choose which technique to use in order to obtain the most diagnostically acceptable films in various clinical situations. The two methods are compared in relation to the rules of shadow casting in the following material.

Principle 1. *X rays should be emitted from as small a point source as possible.* This principle does not pertain to specific intraoral techniques because the dental manufacturer establishes the focal spot size.

Principle 2. *The source-to-object distance should be as long as possible.* Historically, the bisecting-the-angle technique was associated with the use of the short, pointed plastic cone. Using a short distance from the target of the tubehead to the teeth reduces the edge sharpness of the images and increases the magnification of the teeth. The long cone, introduced to be used with the paralleling technique, lengthened the target-object distance in order to improve edge sharpness and reduce magnification. A long cone also should be used with the bisecting-the-angle technique to take advantage of this principle.

Principle 3. *The object-to-film distance should be as short as possible.* The bisecting-the-angle technique satisfies this principle very well because the film packet is placed directly against the teeth. The paralleling method violates this principle somewhat because the films are placed some distance from the teeth. However, the potential loss of edge sharpness and increased magnification is corrected for by the use of a longer cone (16 in.), the use of which takes advantage of shadow-casting Principle 2.

Principles 4 and 5. *The film packet should be placed in a parallel relationship to the teeth and the central ray directed at right angles to the teeth and film.* The paralleling technique was designed to take advantage of these principles in order to eliminate the distortion that was inherent in the images produced by the bisecting-the-angle technique.

The paralleling technique is the generally preferred method of periapical radiography today. In addition to better compliance with shadow-casting principles, there are other advantages when taking the maxillary canine-lateral incisors, premolar, and molar projections. The canine views taken using the bisecting-the-angle technique may result in unacceptable distortion of the root of the canine because of excessive bending of the film packet. This bending is caused by the curved shape of the palate in the anterior region, and when the film is placed, bending of the upper side of the film is difficult to avoid. Maxillary molar and premolar projections taken using the bisecting-the-angle technique may result in superimposition of the zygomatic arch over the roots of the posterior teeth. This is caused by the angled packet position inherent in the bisecting technique with the resulting steep vertical angulations. The paralleling technique corrects for this deficiency by placing the film in a parallel relationship to the long axis of the tooth and aligning the central ray perpendicular to the film, *which is a less steep angle than that used in the bisecting-the-angle technique.* The paralleling method results in the upward projection of the zygomatic arch, providing unobstructed views of the maxillary molar roots (Fig. 54A, B, V-5).

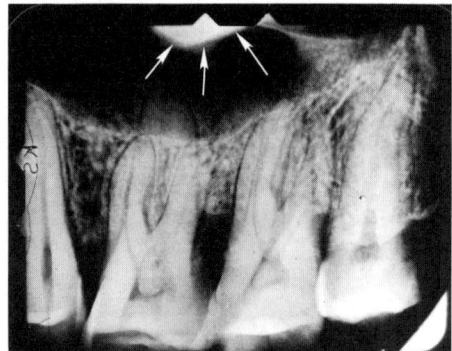

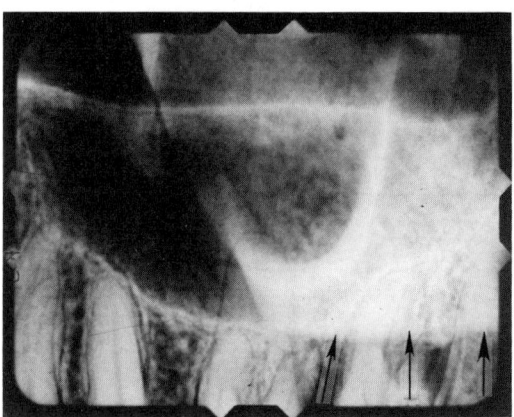

Fig. 54, V-5 Comparison of paralleling and bisecting-the-angle projections for the maxillary molar.

A. Maxillary molars are free of superimposition of zygomatic bone (arrows)—paralleling technique.

B. Maxillary molars with superimposition of zygomatic bone (arrows)—bisecting-the-angle method.

FILM EVALUATION AND ERROR ASSESSMENT

High-quality periapical radiographs should result when the four rules of the paralleling technique are observed. However, variations from the rules can produce film errors. The following criteria serve as guides for evaluating the periapical films in a full mouth series. Although each film is individually critiqued, it is important to consider the entire series for radiographic information before exposing a patient to retakes.

Maxillary Central Incisor Projection

Criteria: A correct film includes both central and lateral incisors in accurate anatomic detail (Fig. 55A, V-5). Retakes may be necessary if the film packet is excessively tipped or angled, or if more than one-half of any lateral incisor is missing (Fig. 55B, V-5). Retakes are also indicated if the film packet is severely bent, teeth extremely elongated, or the incisal one-third of the teeth are cut off (Fig. 55C, V-5).

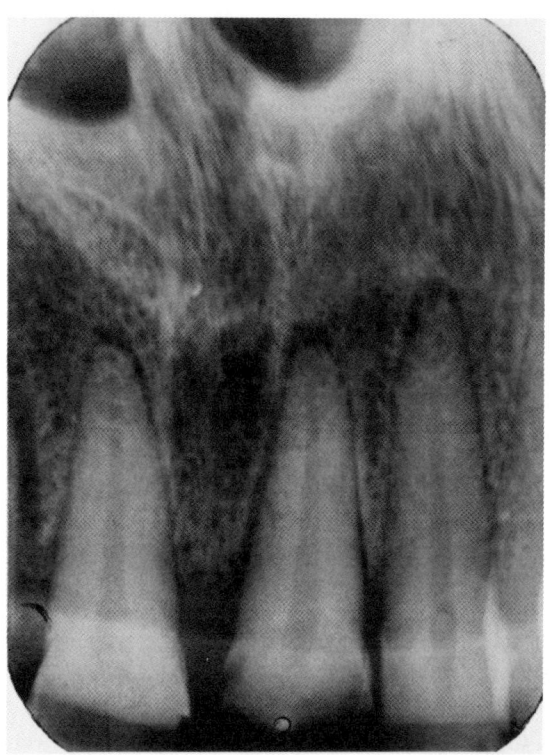

B. Packet placement error: Packet not centered.

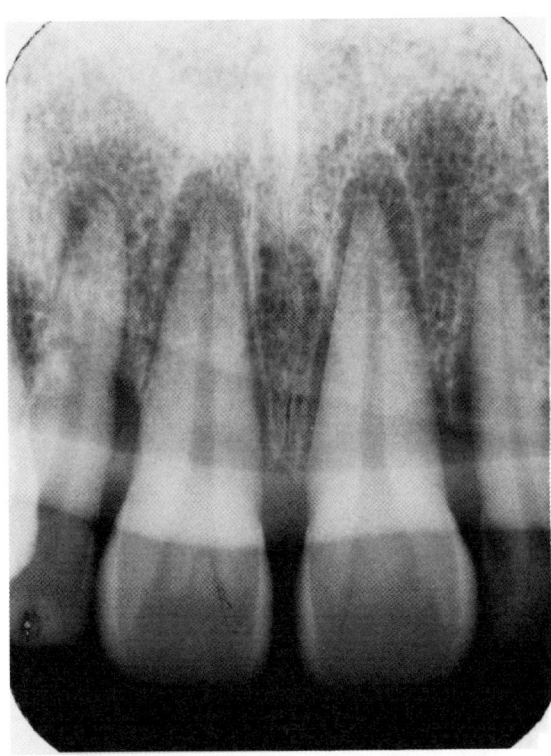

Fig. 55, V-5 Maxillary central incisor projection.
A. Acceptable radiograph: Packet placement, centering, horizontal and vertical angulation are correct.

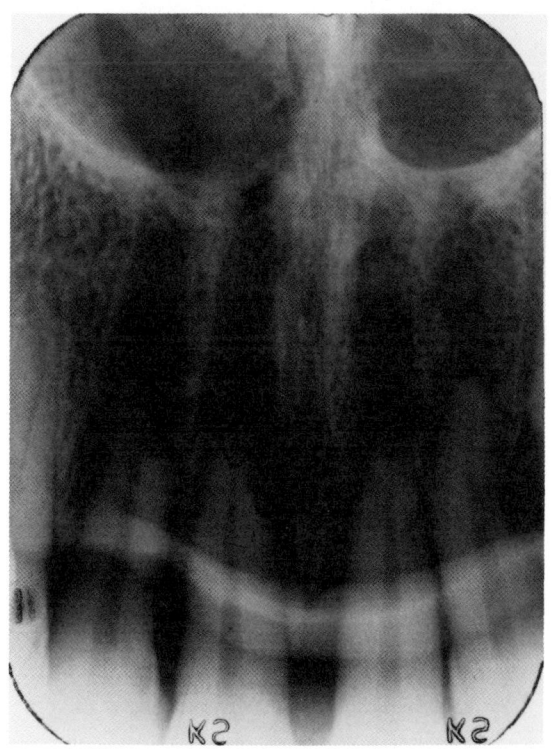

C. Vertical error: Cone angulation too steep.

121

Maxillary Lateral Incisor-Canine Projection

Criteria: A correct film includes all of the lateral incisor and canine, with the interproximal space open (Fig. 56A, V-5). Retakes may be necessary if the apex of either tooth is not visible (Fig. 56B, V-5), if the apices are excessively elongated, or if the incisal one-third is cut off. Excessive horizontal angulation and overlapping of lateral incisor-canine interproximal space also indicates a retake (Fig. 56C, V-5).

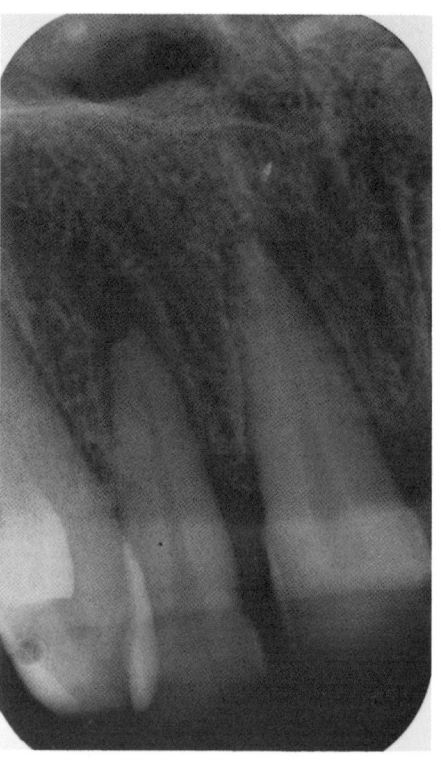

B. Packet placement error: Complete root of canine is not visible.

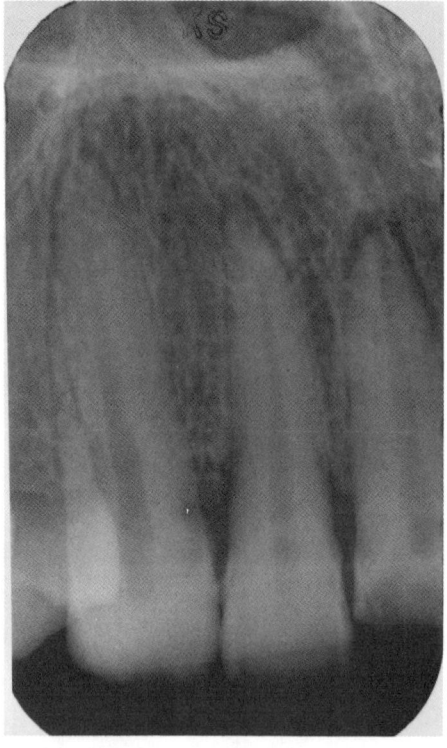

Fig. 56, V-5 Maxillary lateral incisor-canine projection.
A. Acceptable radiograph: Packet placement, centering, horizontal and vertical angulation are correct.

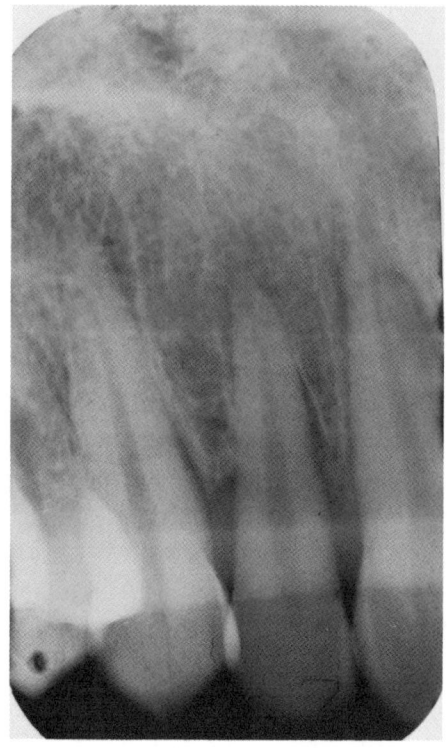

C. Horizontal error: Interproximal space between lateral and canine is not open.

Maxillary Premolar

Criteria: A correct film includes the distal one-half of the canine, both premolars and first molar apices, and variable amounts of the second molar. The interproximal spaces are open between the second premolar and first molar (Fig. 57A, V-5). Retakes may be necessary if the apices of the first and second premolars are not visible, if the apices of the first molar are not visible, if there is severe horizontal overlapping (Fig. 57B, V-5), or if extreme vertical errors are present (Fig. 57C, V-5).

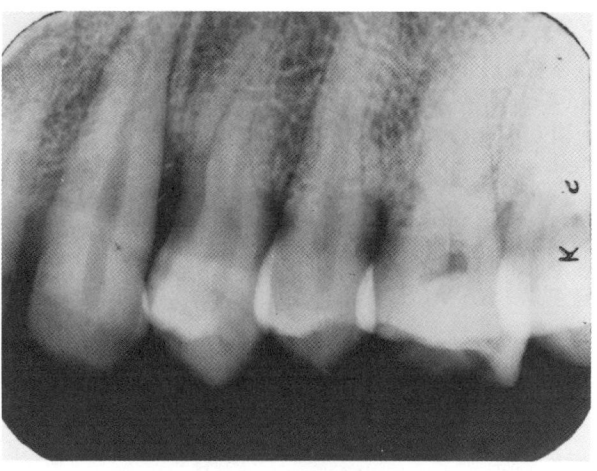

B. Horizontal and vertical error: Cone angulation too mesial and not steep enough.

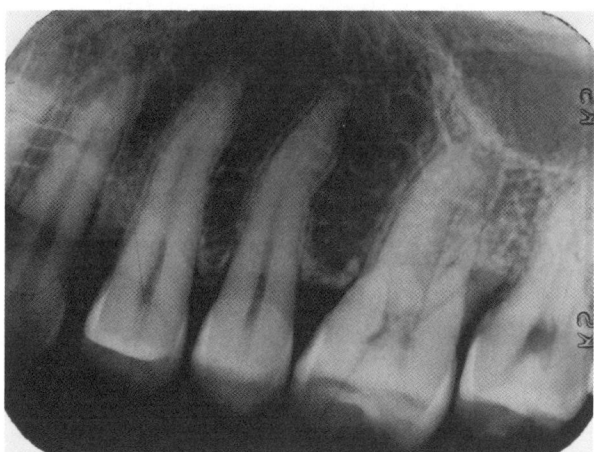

Fig. 57, V-5 Maxillary premolar projection.
A. Acceptable radiograph: Packet placement, centering, horizontal and vertical angulation correct.

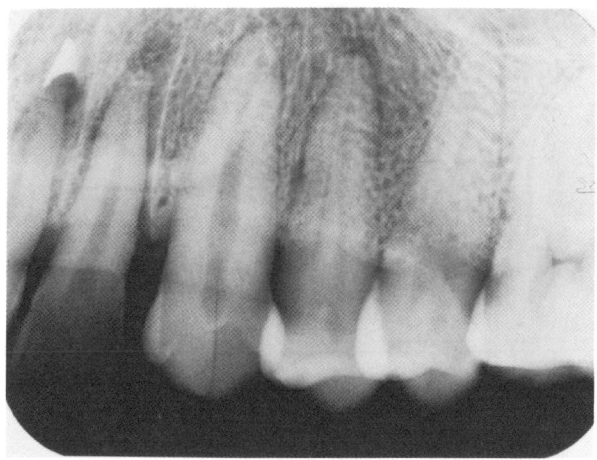

C. Horizontal error: Interproximal spaces not open.

Maxillary Molar

Criteria: A correct film includes most of the first molar and all of the second and third molars with open interproximal spaces (Fig. 58A, V-5). Retakes may be necessary if there are excessive vertical errors (Fig. 58B, V-5), if the apices of the second or third molars are not visible (Fig. 58C, V-5), or if severe horizontal overlapping of the interproximal spaces is present.

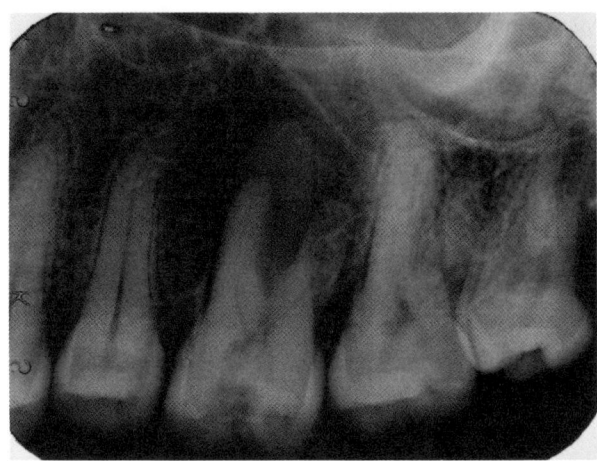

B. Packet placement error: Third molar is not completely visible.

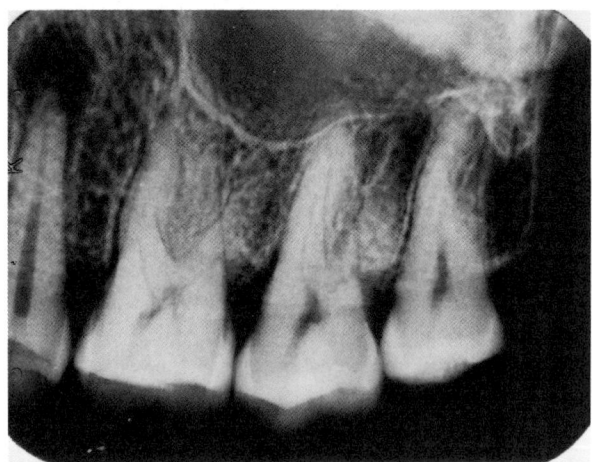

Fig. 58, V-5 Maxillary molar projection.
A. Acceptable radiograph: Packet placement, centering, horizontal and vertical angulation are correct.

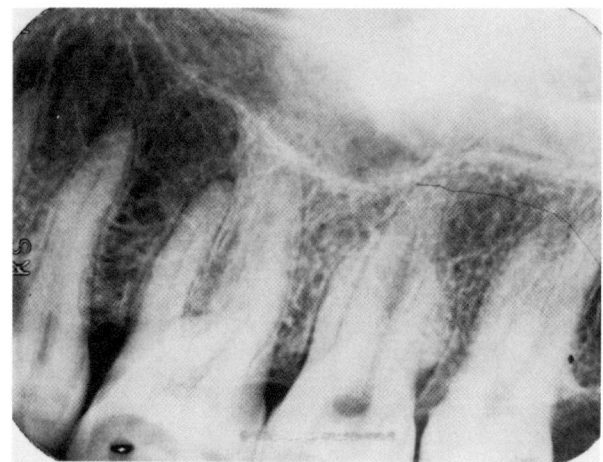

C. Vertical error: Cone angulation is too steep.

Mandibular Central Incisor

Criteria: A correct film shows all of the central and lateral incisors with open interproximal spaces (Fig. 59A, V-5). Retakes may be necessary if there are severe vertical errors, if the apex of either lateral incisor is not visible, or if the incisal one-third is projected off the film (Fig. 59B, V-5).

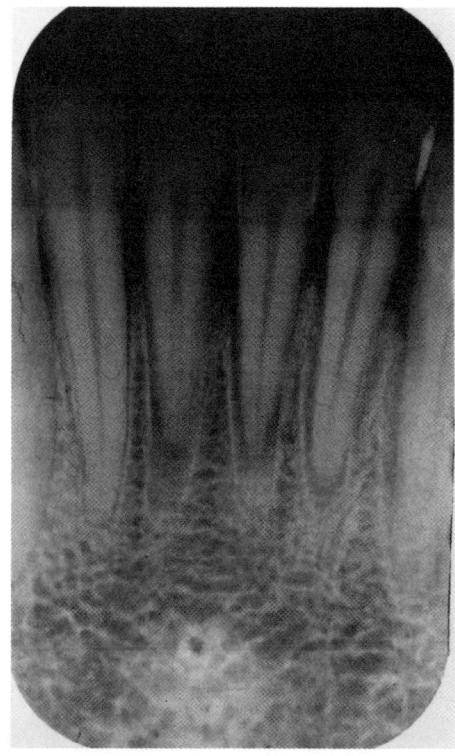 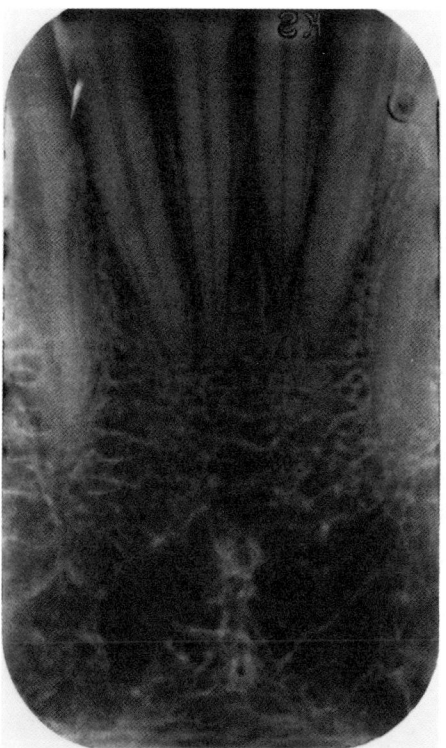

Fig. 59, V-5 Mandibular central incisor projection.
A. Acceptable radiograph: Packet placement, centering, horizontal and vertical angulation are correct.

B. Vertical error: Cone angulation is too steep.

Mandibular Lateral Incisor-Canine

Criteria: A correct film shows the lateral incisor and canine with the interproximal spaces open (Fig. 60A, V-5). Retakes may be necessary if the root apices of the lateral incisor or canine are missing (Fig. 60B, V-5), if there is a severe vertical error, if there is excessive horizontal overlap, or if the incisal one-third of the crowns are not present.

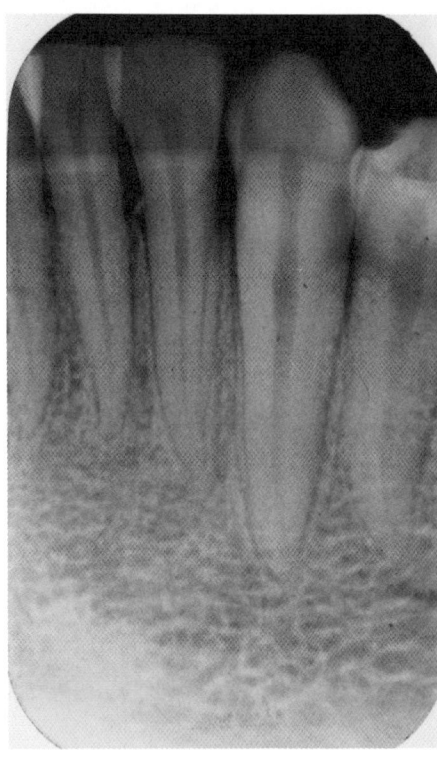 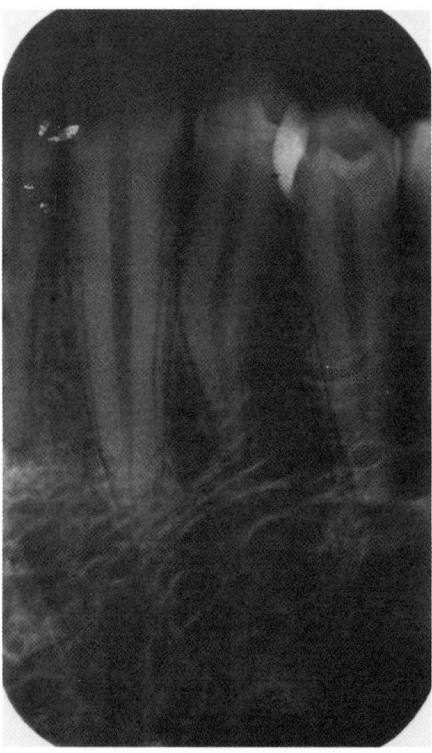

Fig. 60, V-5 Mandibular lateral incisor-canine projection.
A. Acceptable radiograph: Packet placement, centering, horizontal and vertical angulation are correct.

B. Packet placement error: Complete lateral incisor is not visible. Note: Processing error also.

Mandibular Premolar

Criteria: A correct film includes the distal one-half of the canine, the first and second premolars, the first molar, and most of the second molar with open interproximal spaces (Fig. 61A, V-5). Retakes may be necessary if the apices of the first and second premolars or molar apices are not visible (Fig. 61B, V-5), if there are excessive vertical errors (Fig. 61C, V-5), or if severe horizontal overlapping is present.

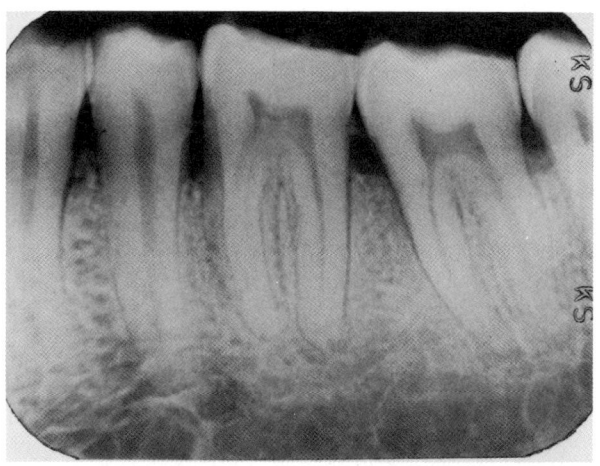

B. Packet placement error: Complete first premolar is not visible.

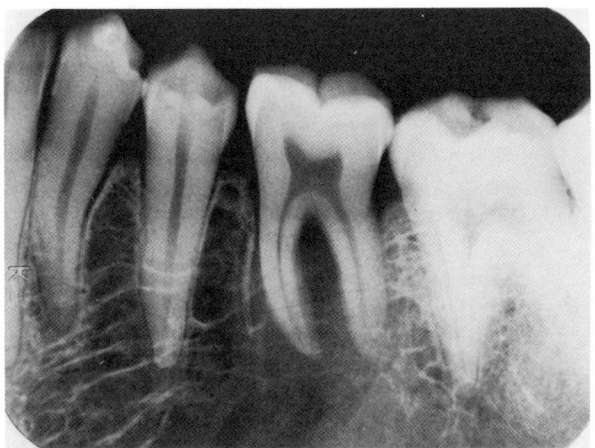

Fig. 61, V-5 Mandibular premolar projection.

A. Acceptable radiograph: Packet placement, centering, horizontal and vertical angulation are correct.

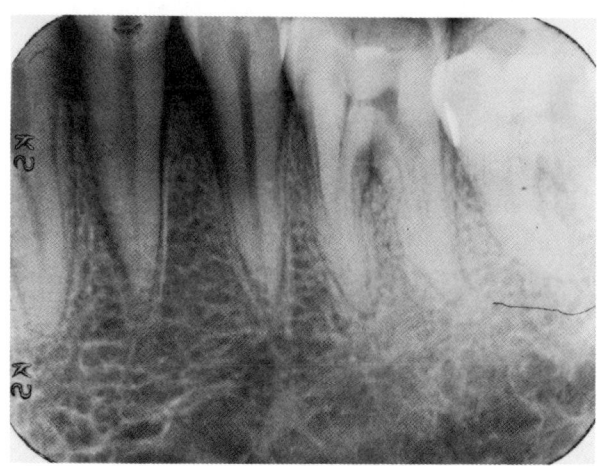

C. Vertical error: Cone angulation is too steep.

Mandibular Molar

Criteria: A correct film shows most (if not all) of the first molar and all of the second and third molars with open interproximal spaces (Fig. 62A, V-5). Retakes may be necessary if any molar apex is not visible (Fig. 62B, V-5), if there is severe horizontal overlapping or extreme vertical error, or if the coronal one-third is projected off the film.

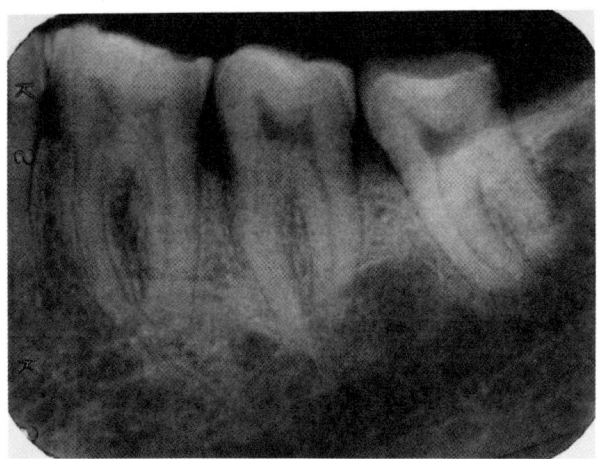 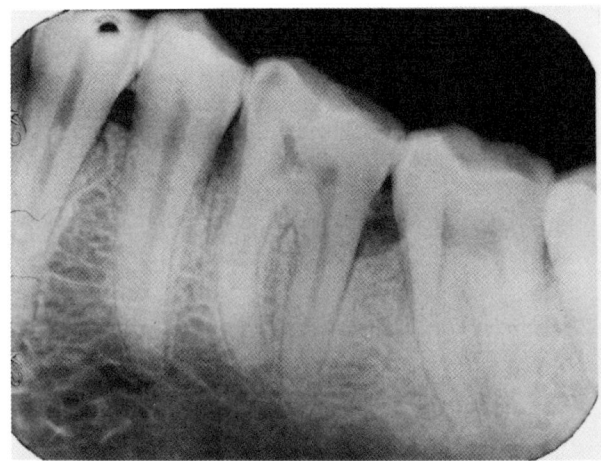

Fig. 62, V-5 Mandibular molar projection.
A. Acceptable radiograph: Packet placement, centering, horizontal and vertical angulation are correct.

B. Packet placement error: Apices of all molars are not visible.

Premolar Bitewing

Criteria: A correct film shows the distal one-half of both canines, crowns of the premolars, first molars, and most of the second molars with open interproximal spaces and equal distribution of the maxillary and mandibular teeth (Fig. 63A, V-5). Retakes may be necessary if the distal half of the canines is not visible (Fig. 63B, V-5), if there is extreme horizontal overlapping or unequal distribution of maxillary and mandibular teeth (Fig. 63C, V-5), or if distorted crowns are present.

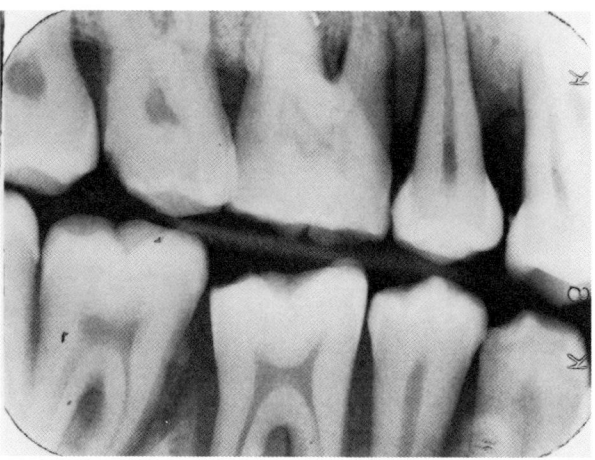

B. Packet placement error: Distal halves of canines are not visible.

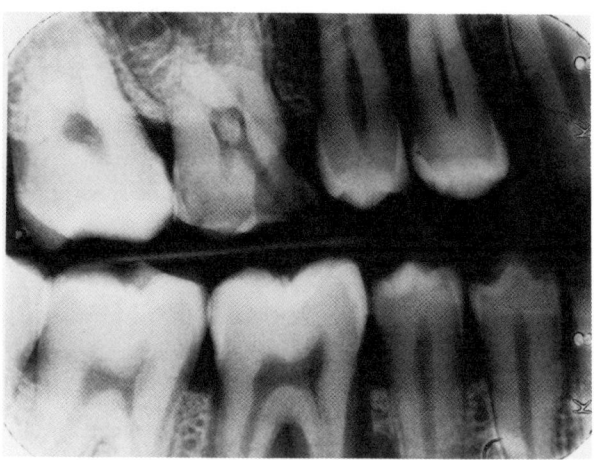

Fig. 63, V-5 Premolar bitewing projection.

A. Acceptable radiograph: Packet placement, centering, horizontal and vertical angulation are correct.

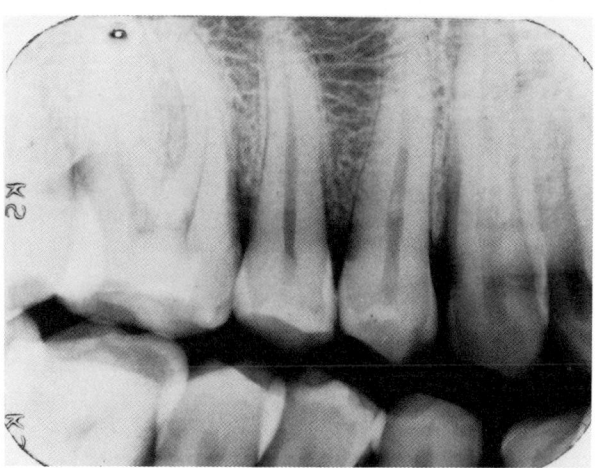

C. Vertical error: Cone is not at +10° or the packet slipped.

Molar Bitewing

Criteria: A correct film includes all of the molar crowns with equal distribution of maxillary and mandibular teeth with open interproximal spaces (Fig. 64A, V-5). Retakes may be necessary if errors are similar to the premolar errors (Fig. 64B, C, V-5).

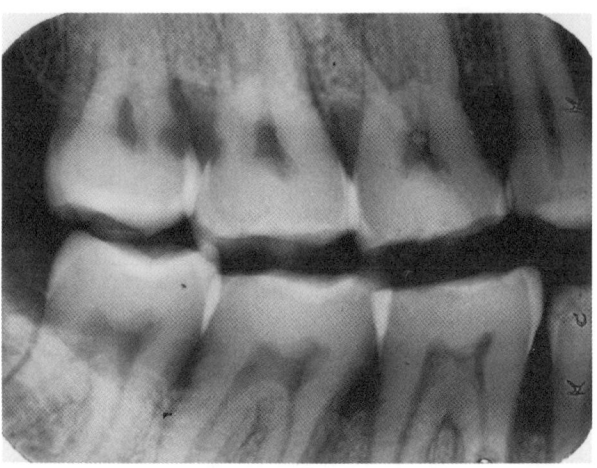

B. Horizontal error: Interproximal spaces are overlapped.

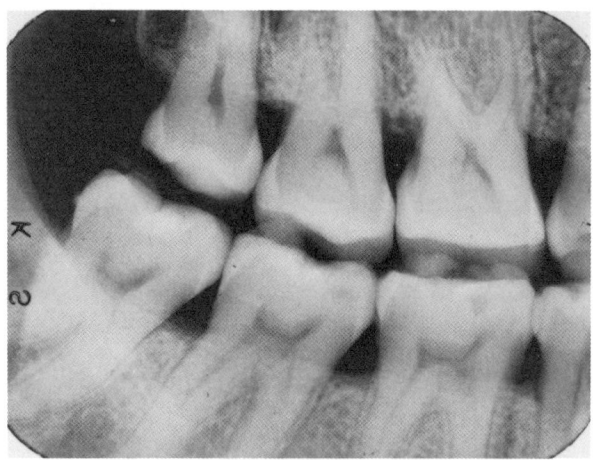

Fig. 64, V-5 Molar bitewing projection.
A. Acceptable radiograph: Packet placement, centering, horizontal and vertical angulation are correct.

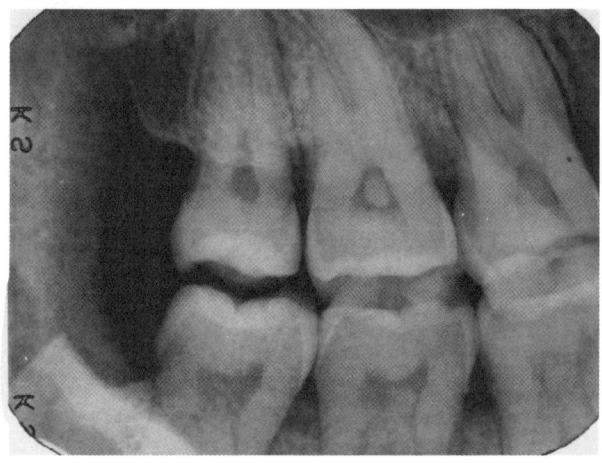

C. Packet placement error: Occlusal plane not centered.

BIBLIOGRAPHY

Eastman Kodak Company. *X-Rays in Dentistry*. Rochester, N.Y.: Radiology Markets Division, 1985.

Frommer, H. H. *Radiology for Dental Auxiliaries*. 4th ed. St. Louis: C. V. Mosby Co., 1987.

Langland, O. E.; Langlais, R. P.; Sippy, F. H.; and Williamson, G. *Radiology for Dental Hygienists and Dental Assistants*. Springfield, Ill.: Charles C. Thomas, 1988.

Section 5

Examination

In a few words, phrases, or sentences, answer the following questions. Use a separate sheet of paper.

1. Define intraoral radiographic technique.
2. Define extraoral radiographic technique.
3. List the five shadow-casting principles.
4. Which movement of the tubehead establishes the vertical angulation?
5. Which movement of the tubehead establishes the horizontal angulation?
6. Why was the paralleling periapical technique introduced?
7. List the four rules of procedure for the paralleling technique.
8. In the paralleling technique, what is the effect on the radiographic image of the use of vertical angulation that is too steep?
9. What is the effect on the radiographic image of the use of incorrect horizontal angulation?
10. What is the result on the radiographic image of incorrect centering of the exposure field on the film?
11. Why is the end of the Stabe removed for use in the mandibular premolar and molar projections?
12. List the four rules of procedure for the bisecting-the-angle technique.
13. In the bisecting-the-angle technique, what is the effect on the radiographic image of the use of a vertical angle that is
    a. Too steep?
    b. Not steep enough?
14. What are the advantages of the paralleling periapical technique?
15. Describe packet placement, vertical angulation, and horizontal angulation used for obtaining:
    a. The premolar bitewing radiograph.
    b. The molar bitewing radiograph.
16. What patient exposure reduction is achieved when using the Precision Instrument?

Supplemental Techniques

This section describes the procedures for obtaining extraoral and intraoral supplemental projections. These radiographs may be indicated when standard intraoral films do not provide sufficient information to make a diagnosis or when patients have certain unusual clinical problems.

OBJECTIVES

1. To discuss panoramic radiographic techniques and list their uses.
2. To list the steps used to position a patient correctly for a panorex radiograph.
3. To discuss cephalometric radiographic technique and to state its principal use.
4. To discuss the lateral oblique mandible radiographic technique and to state its use.
5. To discuss the radiographic technique used to demonstrate the temporomandibular joint.
6. To list the indications for taking third molar disto-oblique radiographs and to give the methods used for maxillary and mandibular projections.
7. To give the indications for taking occlusal radiographs and to discuss the methods used when taking topographical and cross-sectional occlusal projections.

EXTRAORAL

Panoramic Radiography

The panoramic radiograph is the most routinely obtained extraoral film in the dental office. It is exposed using special x-ray equipment. Images are recorded when the x-ray tubehead and film rotate on a fixed axis around the patient. Prior to exposure, the film is loaded into a cassette. The use of cassettes with intensifying screens considerably reduces radiation exposure to the patient. Rather than relying on 18 individual intraoral radiographs, the dentist can look at a panoramic film that shows the entire dental arches and surrounding structures on one film. In certain cases this can be an important diagnostic advantage. Exposure times for panoramic methods are preset and are usually from 15 to 22 sec. The panoramic film is easier to obtain than a full series of intraoral radiographs and causes little or no discomfort to the patient. Processing procedures follow the same rules as for intraoral film and can be accomplished using either automatic or manual methods. Indications for obtaining panoramic films are (1) to provide a survey film for edentulous patients, (2) to assess growth and development, and (3) when intraoral radiographs are impossible to obtain, such as for trauma patients, patients with severe gagging problems, handicapped patients, or small children. With reference to film quality, panoramic images do not possess the sharp resolution or detail one sees when viewing intraoral films. This is because during a pan-

oramic exposure, motion of the tubehead and film are necessary to obtain this projection and because cassettes with intensifying screens are used (Fig. 1A, B, V-6).

Fig. 2, V-6 shows a patient correctly positioned for a Panorex and a resulting radiograph. The head is extended upward and forward, allowing the patient's chin to rotate downward and into the chin rest or focal plane of the machine. The use of an angled sponge cushion is recommended to straighten the patient's back. The patient's head is then positioned with the occlusal plane parallel to the floor. The chin rest can be locked into position. The sagittal plane of the patient should be perpendicular to the floor, and the patient should be instructed to look straight ahead. After these minor adjustments in position have been made, the pancentric headholders are moved into place to further center and stabilize the head. Next, the film is centered beside the jaws by raising or lowering the film carriage and tubehead. This has been correctly done when the number on the chin-rest post matches the corresponding number on the scale located on the vertical panorex case behind the patient. The teeth are slightly separated by placing a cotton roll between the central incisors. This prevents overlapping of the maxillary and mandibular anterior teeth on the radiograph.

Another type of panoramic equipment is available as shown in Fig. 3, V-6. Slight differences in the image are noted, but the diagnostic information provided and principles of operation are similar.

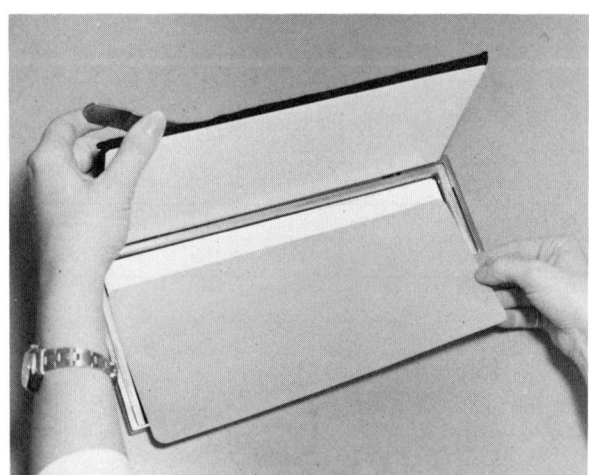

Fig. 1, V-6 Cassettes and film.
    A. Cassette and film for Panorex.

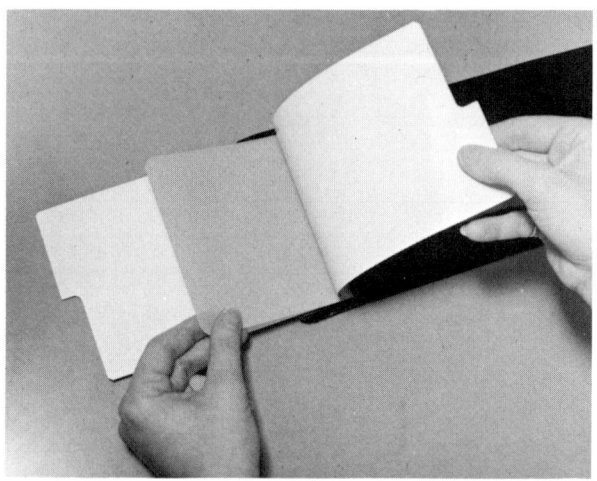

B. Flexible cassette and film for Panelipse.

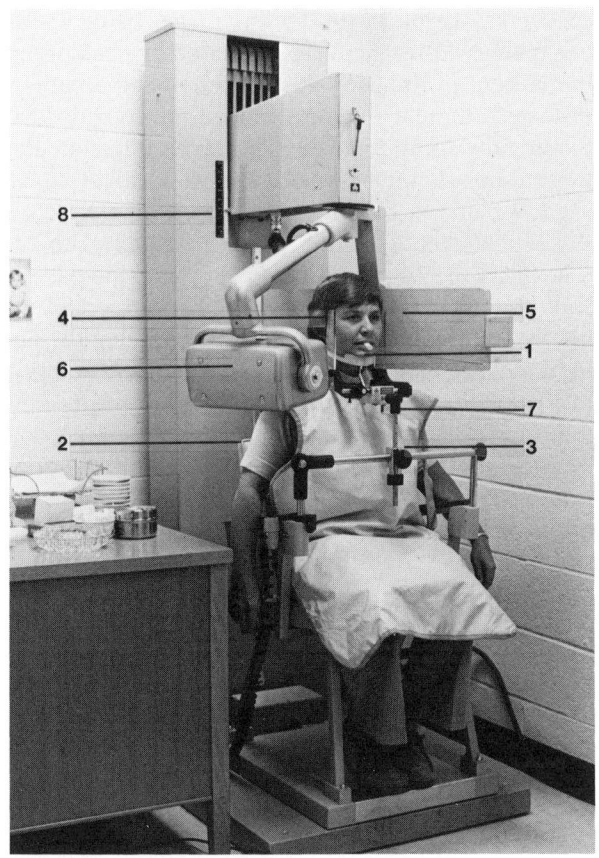

Fig. 2, V-6

A. Patient positioned for Panorex radiograph. (1) Chin rest, (2) angled sponge, (3) chin rest lock, (4) pan-centric head holder, (5) film carriage, (6) tubehead, (7) chin-rest post, and (8) vertical scale.

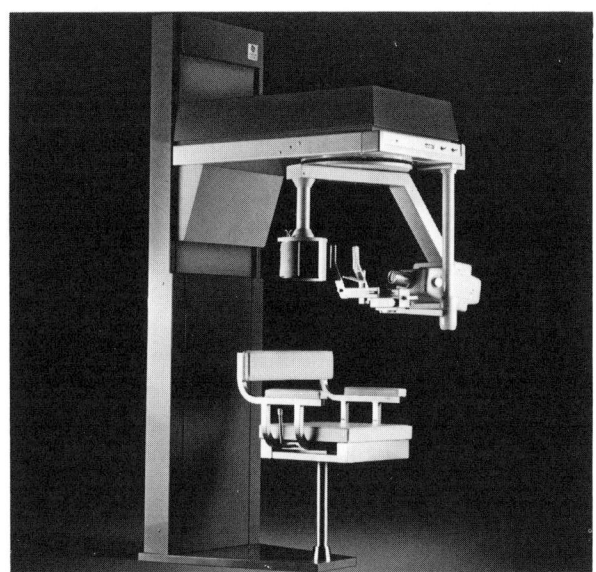

Fig. 3, V-6

A. Panelipse x-ray machine. *(Courtesy of General Electric Co., Milwaukee, WI)*

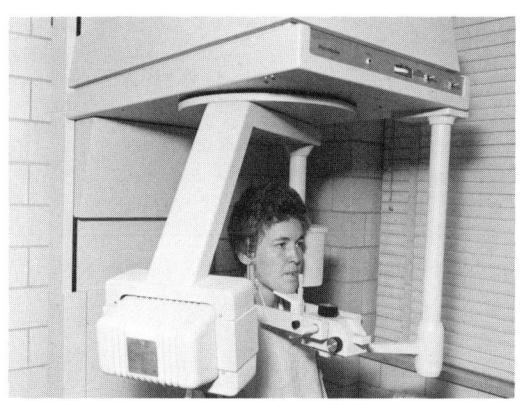

B. Patient seated for Panelipse radiograph.

B. Resulting radiograph.

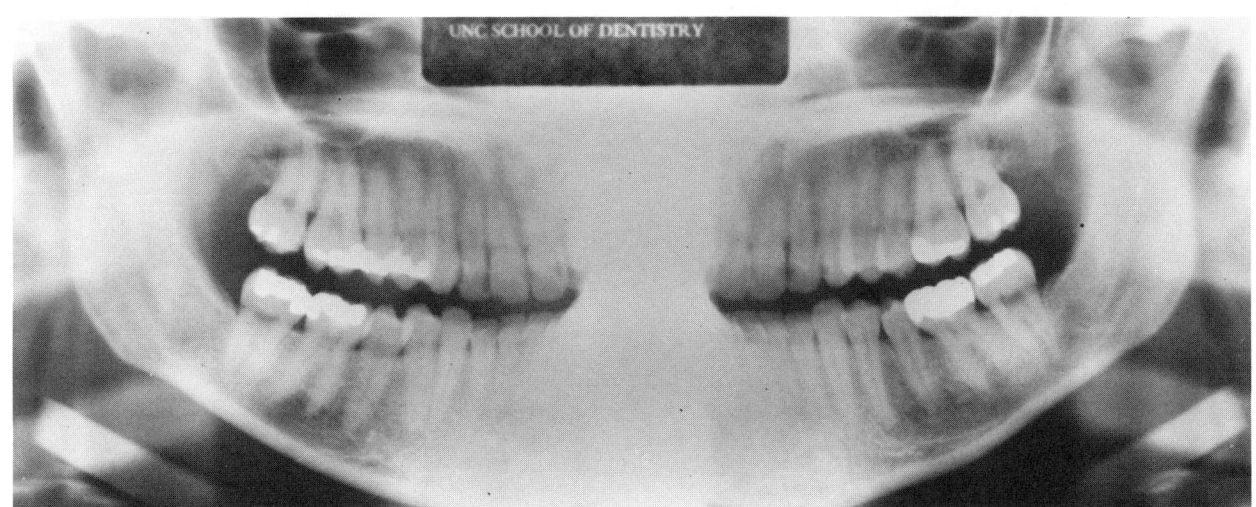

Cephalometric Radiography

The cephalometric radiograph provides information used when evaluating the orthodontic or pediatric patient. Because patients undergoing orthodontic treatment may require a series of cephalometric radiographs during the course of growth and development, standardized procedures are needed to make these comparisons. The first and most important requirement is that the patient's head be placed in the same position for each exposure. To accomplish this, a head-holding device is used, the *cephalostat*, which incorporates the use of ear posts to position the patient in identical positions for each film (Fig. 4A, B, V-6).

The equipment installation is standardized with a 60-in. distance between the x-ray source and the mid-sagittal plane of the patient. The source can be an intraoral dental tubehead mounted for cephalometric procedures (Fig. 5A, B, V-6) or a larger medical x-ray machine (Fig. 5C, V-6). Both are capable of exposing cephalometric radiographs, but the medical unit is capable of producing images using shorter exposure times. Films are obtained by positioning the patient in the cephalostat and after the patient is seated, the ear rods are moved into position by rotating the appropriate handle. Once completed, the measurement of the distance from the patient's mid-sagittal plane to the film is indicated on a scale on the cephalostat. This dimension is usually 11.5 cm (Fig. 5D, V-6). With the ear rods in place, the patient should be instructed to look straight ahead, establishing the natural head position. To ensure that the patient will not move, the forehead stabilizer is moved into position as shown. Soft tissue profiles representing the natural appearance of the patient must also be included on the film. This is accomplished by placing a wedge filter on the x-ray tubehead in order to absorb a portion of the x-ray beam. The facial soft tissues are then underexposed and the profile appears on the film. Figs. 4, 5, V-6 demonstrate cephalometric procedures and an example of a cephalometric radiograph is shown in Figure 5E, V-6.

Cephalometric Technique

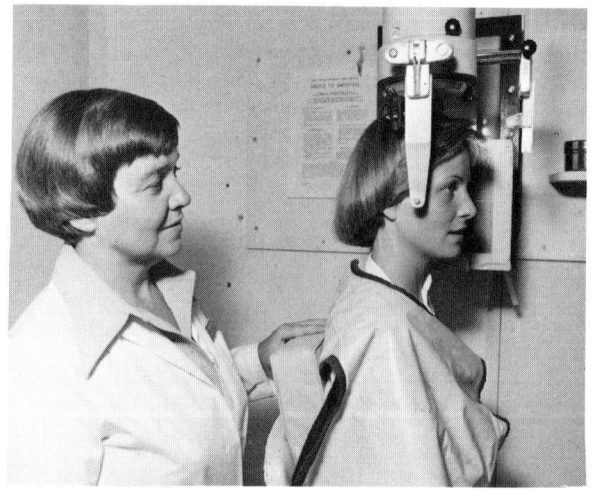

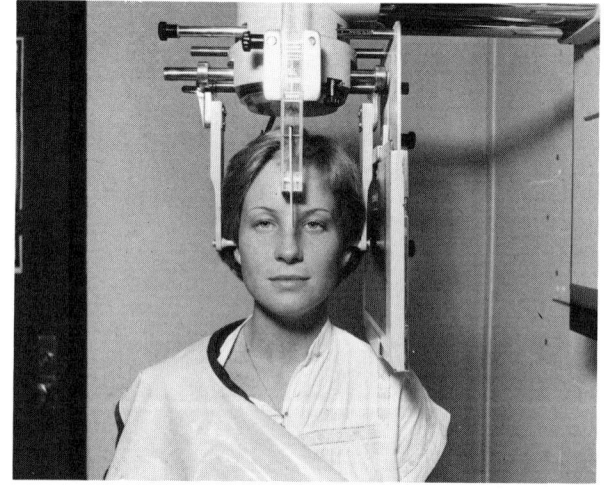

Fig. 4, V-6 Cephalometric technique.
A. Patient being seated for cephalometric projection.

B. Patient positioning with ear rods in place.

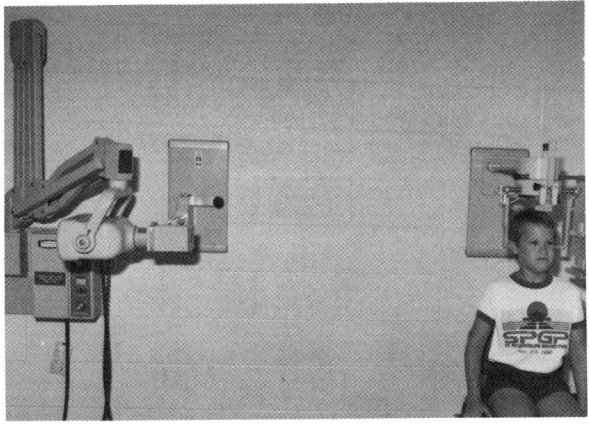

Fig. 5, V-6

A. Cephalometric setup with intraoral x-ray equipment for patient in sitting position.

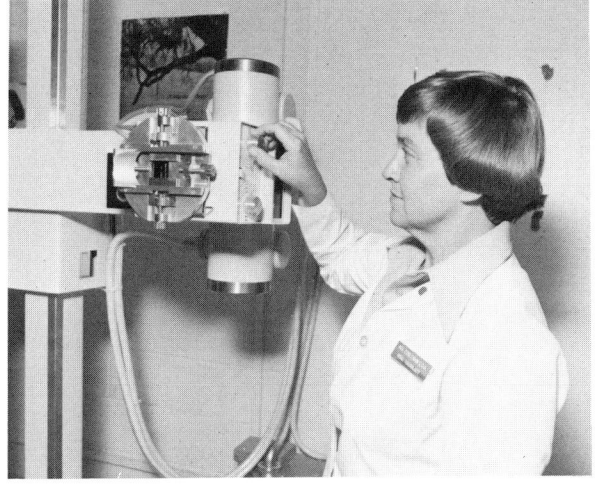

C. Collimation of x-ray beam.

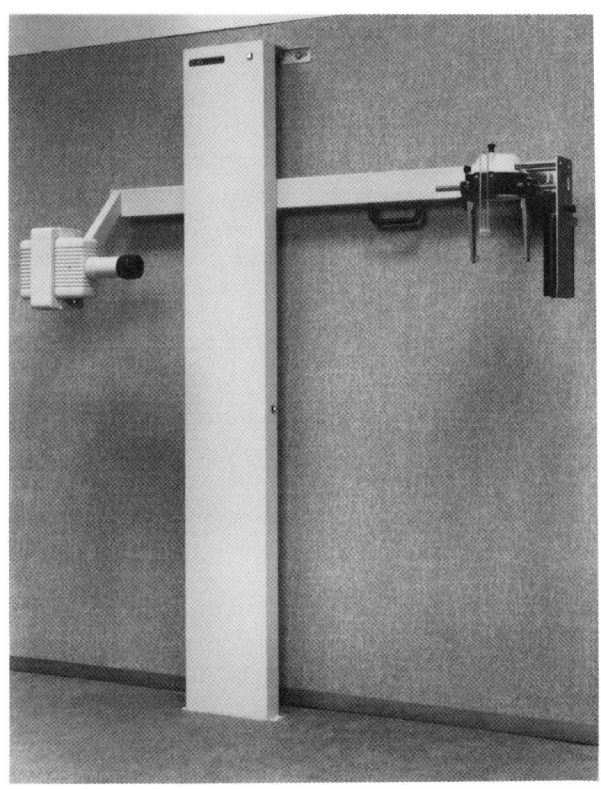

B. Cephalometric setup with intraoral equipment for patient in standing position. *(Courtesy of Gendex Corp., Milwaukee, WI)*

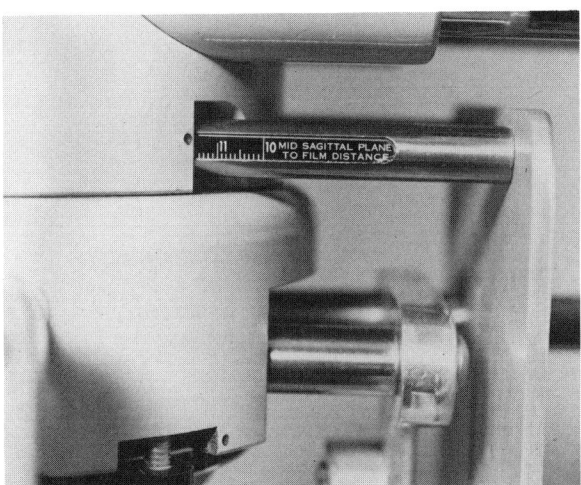

D. Standard 11.5 cm mid-sagittal plane-to-film distance.

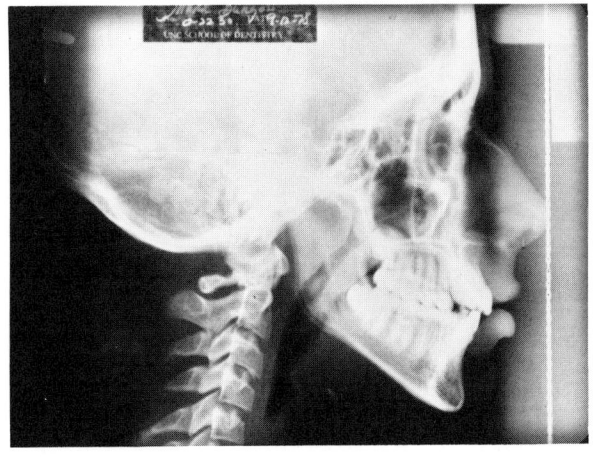

E. Cephalometric radiograph.

The Lateral Oblique Mandible

The lateral oblique mandible is one of the more easily obtained extraoral projections. Patients should experience little or no discomfort during the exposure of this film. Equipment needed includes a 5-in. × 12-in. or 5-in. × 7-in. cassette with film and an x-ray unit. In Fig. 6, V-6 the intraoral unit serves as the x-ray source. This unit is similar to the type found in most dental offices. Notice that a short cone replaces the 16-in. cone. For this projection, use of a longer cone restricts the field size to less than is needed. The patient is seated and then turned in the chair so that the cassette can rest between the head rest and lateral side of the face. The patient's midsagittal plane is aligned to be parallel to the plane of the cassette. To eliminate motion, the cassette should rest on the patient's shoulder. The occlusal plane should be perpendicular to the plane of the film. The x-ray cone is directed 25 degrees to the negative (aiming upward) with the x-ray field centered to the ramus of the mandible. Figure 7A, B, V-6 demonstrates a Franklin headstand. Advantages to using this equipment are that it provides a special tray for holding the cassette; it can record images with faster exposure times; and it has an adjustable field size to accommodate the area being exposed. The tray is referred to as a "bucky tray" and has a grid that serves to absorb scatter radiation as it exits the patient during the exposure. This factor improves image contrast.

Indications for obtaining this projection are usually of a supplemental nature. For instance, radiolucencies and radiopacities visualized in initial radiographs can be reexposed using a different angulation. This projection can be useful when artifacts in panoramic radiographs obscure patient anatomy. Figure 8, V-6 shows a lateral oblique mandible radiograph. The area demonstrated on the radiograph extends from the canine region posteriorly to the mandibular body and ramus.

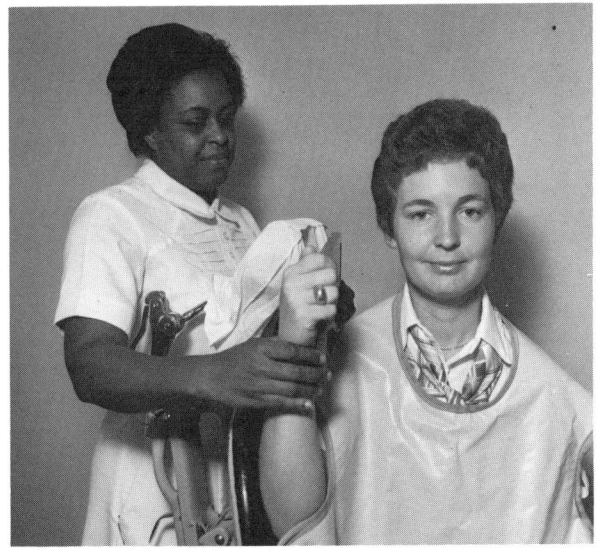

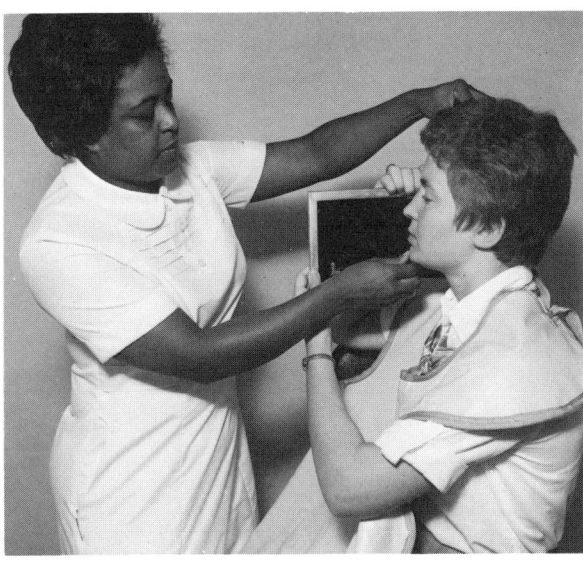

Fig. 6, V-6 Lateral oblique mandible projection using dental x-ray machine.

A. Cassette rests on patient's shoulder.

B. The mandible is slightly extended.

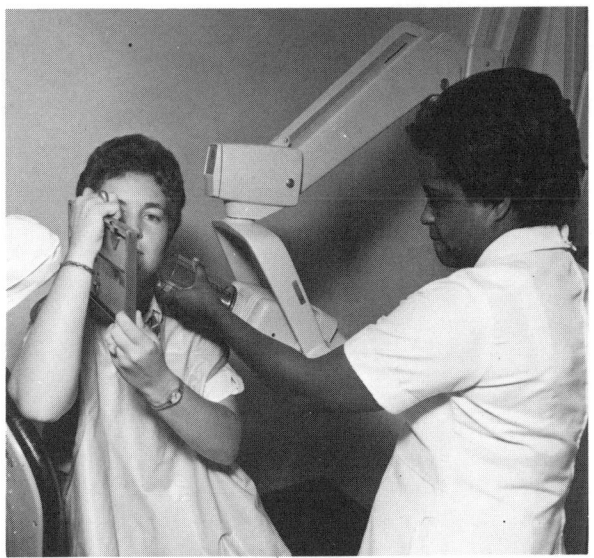

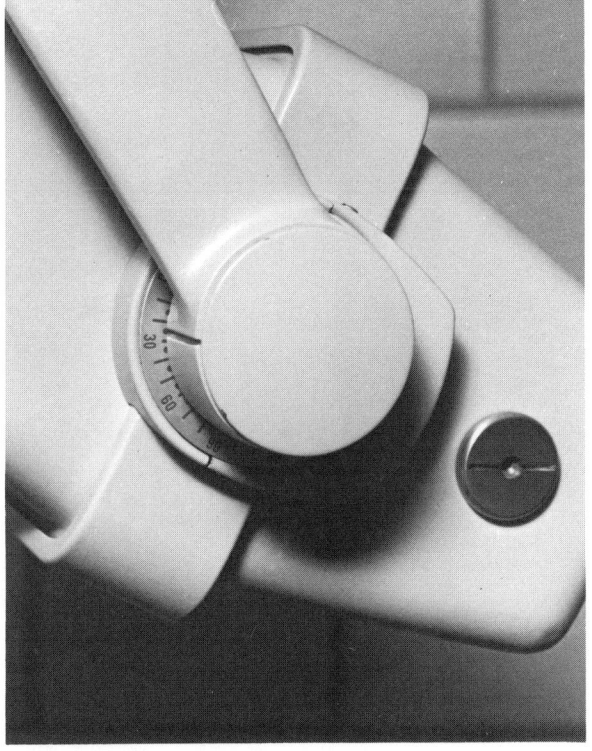

C. The cone is directed toward the mandible.

D. 25-degree negative angulation.

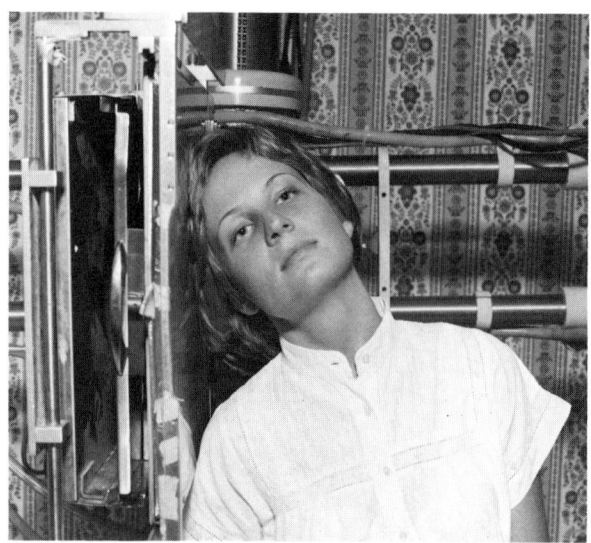

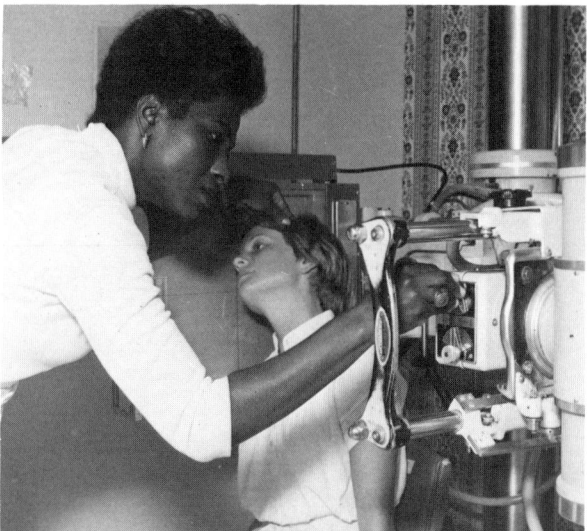

Fig. 7, V-6 Lateral oblique mandible projection using medical x-ray machine.

    A. The head is flexed laterally toward the film.

B. X rays are directed perpendicular to film.

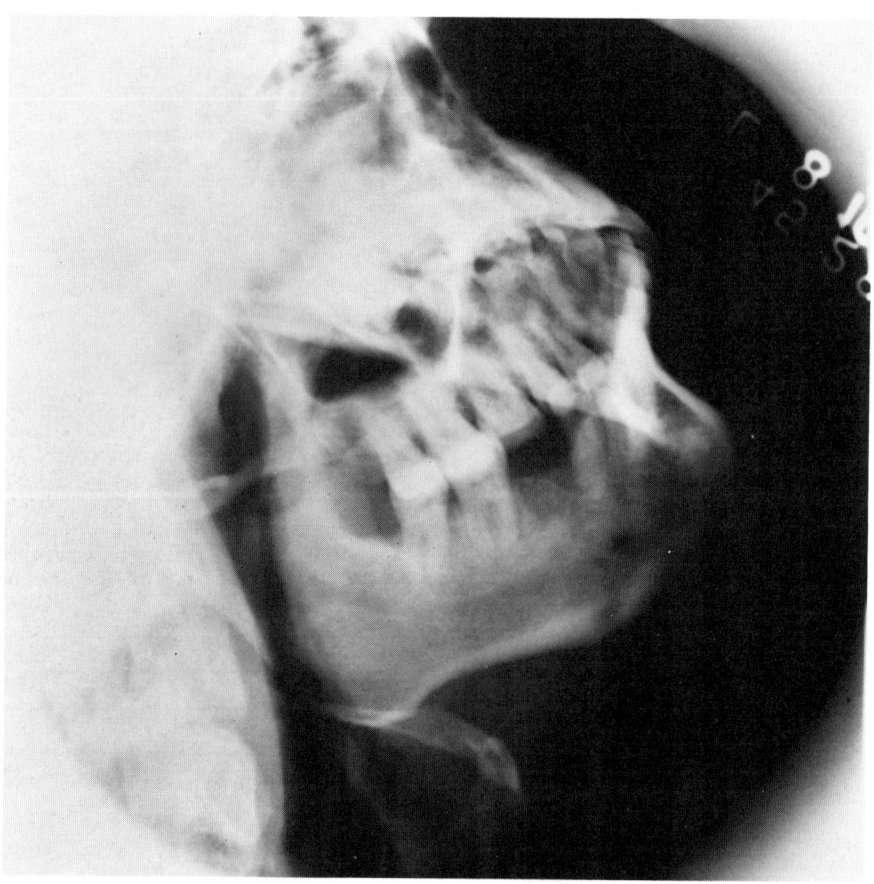

Fig. 8, V-6 Lateral oblique mandible radiograph.

Temporomandibular Joint Radiography

Patients who complain of pain or clicking in the temporomandibular joint or those who have sustained a blow to the mandible may require radiographs of the joint. This projection is exposed with the patient in the erect position. A cassette loaded with screen film is used, and the side of the patient being radiographed is positioned against the film. The sagittal plane of the patient is parallel to the film. The x-ray cone is directed from the opposite side, and the vertical angulation is aligned at 30 degrees to the positive (aiming downward). The horizontal angu-

lation is established at a right angle to the sagittal plane. The point of entry of the x-ray beam is approximately 3 in. above the ear and is fixed so as to direct the beam to exit at the joint being radiographed. Figure 9A, B, V-6 show the patient positioning and cone alignment used for this technique, using a medical x-ray unit. An example of a temporomandibular joint radiograph is shown in Figure 9C, V-6.

This projection can be accomplished using a dental x-ray machine. Several devices are available that position the patient when using a standard dental machine.

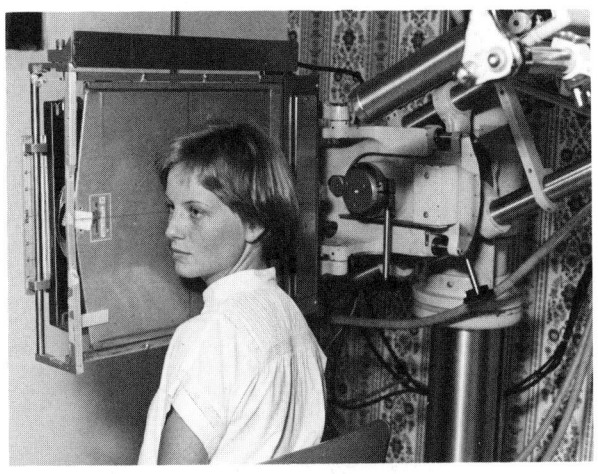

Fig. 9, V-6 Temporomandibular joint projection.
A. Closed-mouth position.

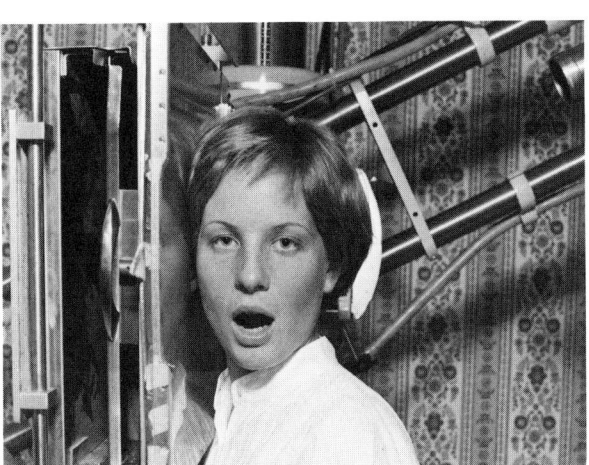

B. Open-mouth position.

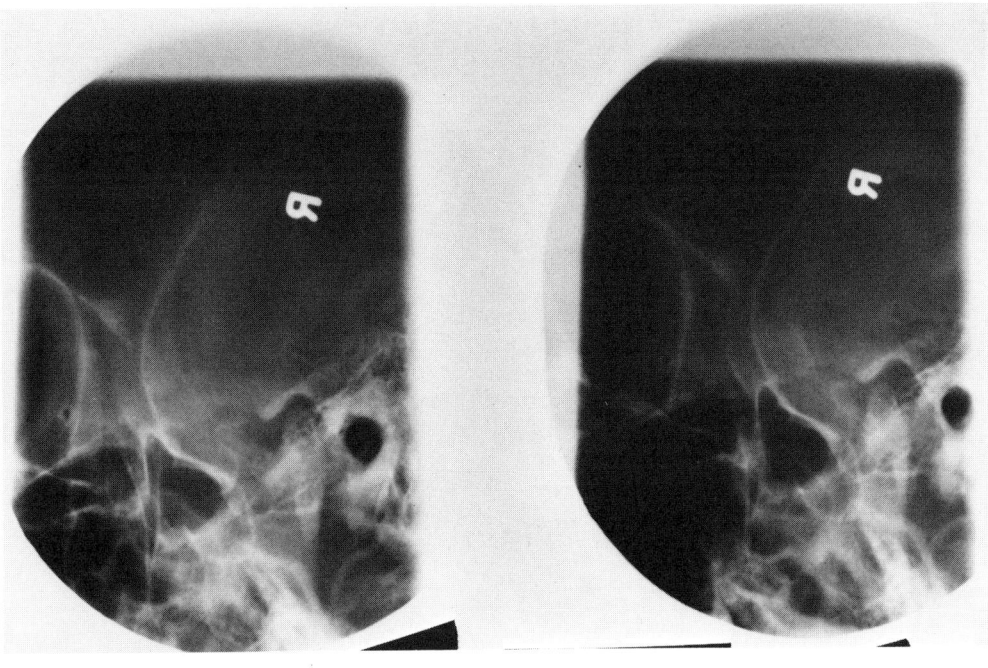

C. Resulting radiograph (left, closed; right, open).

INTRAORAL

Third Molar Disto-Oblique Technique

The third molar disto-oblique technique is used to obtain radiographs of third molars that are impacted in the jaws or when patients are unable to tolerate the film packet in the usual molar position. The top radiographs in Figs. 10, 11, V-6 do not include the entire third molars. The method described below enables the dental assistant to project these teeth onto the film when this clinical problem occurs.

MAXILLA. For maxillary third molars, the film packet is placed as far posteriorly as possible. After aligning the cone as would be usual for a normal molar projection, the horizontal angulation is shifted 5–10 degrees from the distal, and the vertical angulation is increased 10 degrees, or an angle that is steeper from above (Fig. 10, V-6).

MANDIBLE. For mandibular third molars, the film packet is placed as far posteriorly as possible. After aligning the cone as would be usual for a normal molar projection, the horizontal angulation is shifted 10 degrees from the distal. No change is made in the vertical angulation (Fig. 11, V-6).

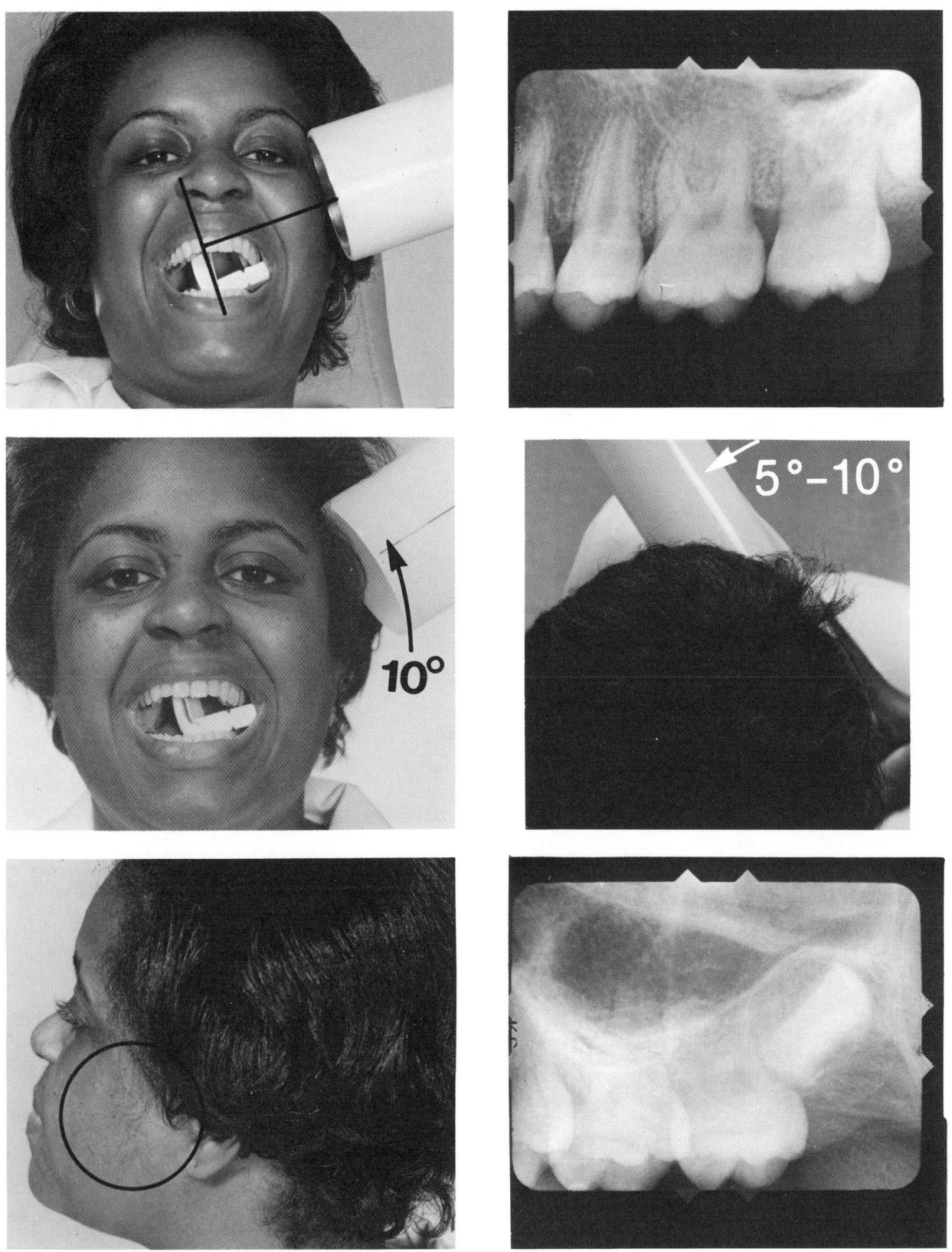

Fig. 10, V-6 Maxillary third molar disto-oblique.

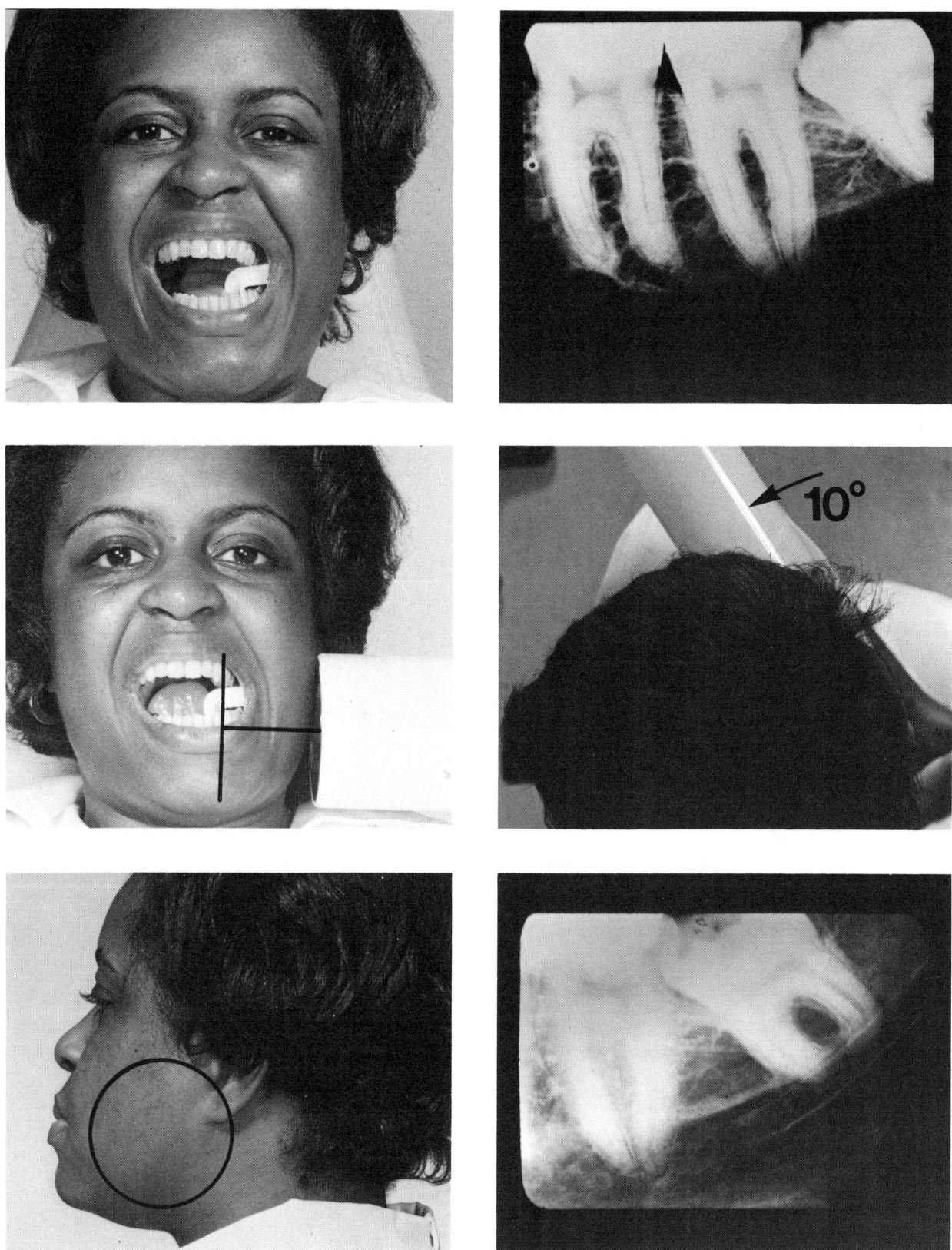

Fig. 11, V-6 Mandibular third molar disto-oblique.

OCCLUSAL RADIOGRAPHY

Occlusal radiographs are taken with the film packets placed along the occlusal plane. They are used to provide wider views of the jaws or for children in whom placement of periapical films is impossible. An occlusal size film is normally used, but for small patients a #2 size packet may be indicated.

MAXILLARY TOPOGRAPHICAL PROJECTION. To obtain the topographical projection of the maxillary anterior area, the film packet is placed between the upper and lower teeth with the tube side of the film facing upward. The patient is asked to close on the film, and this holds the film in place. With the film packet (and occlusal plane) adjusted to be parallel to the floor, an angle of 60–65 degrees is established. The horizontal angulation is established with the central ray passing through the interproximal space between the central incisors. The point of entry of the x-ray beam is the bridge of the nose (Fig. 12, V-6).

MANDIBULAR TOPOGRAPHICAL PROJECTION. This film shows the anterior mandible. To obtain this projection, the film packet is placed between the upper and lower teeth with the tube side of the packet downward. The patient holds the film in position by biting on the packet. With the occlusal plane (and film) positioned parallel to the floor, the vertical angulation is established at −55 degrees (aiming upward). The horizontal angulation is set with the central ray directed through the interproximal space between the central incisors (Fig. 13, V-6).

MANDIBULAR CROSS-SECTIONAL PROJECTION. The mandibular cross-sectional radiograph is used to show the mandible as seen from below and to study the floor of the mouth for salivary stones. After placing the film along the occlusal surfaces and having the patient close on the packet, the cone is directed from below at right angles to the film (Fig. 14, V-6).

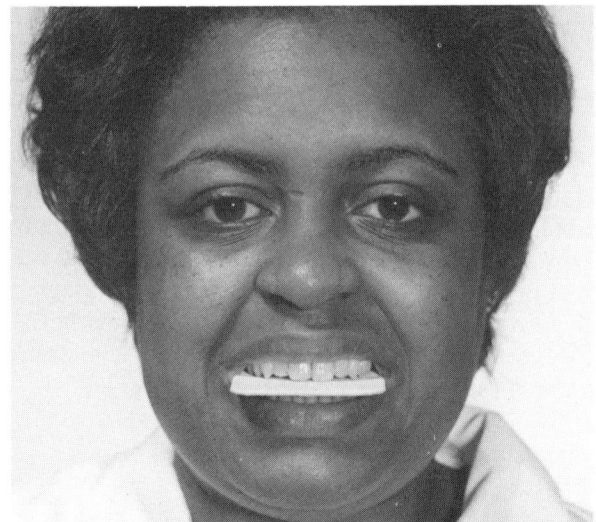

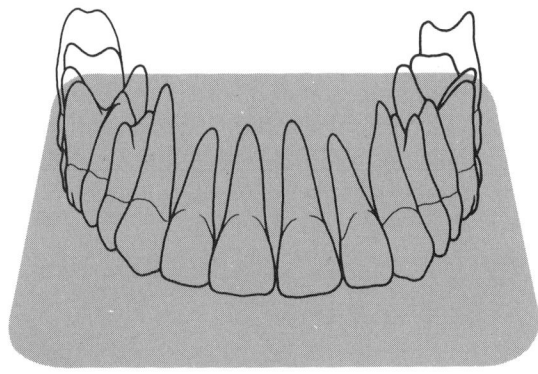

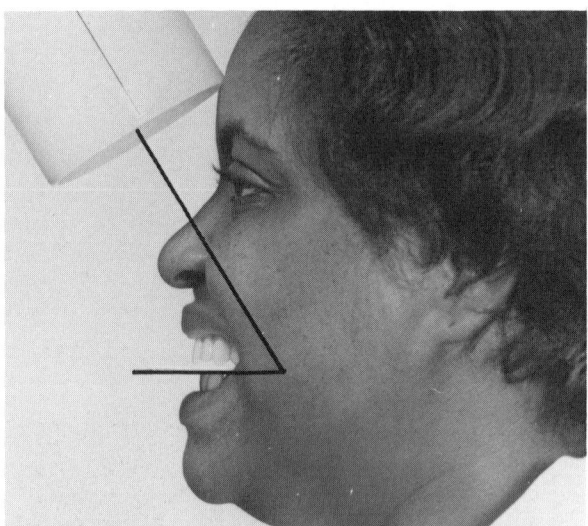

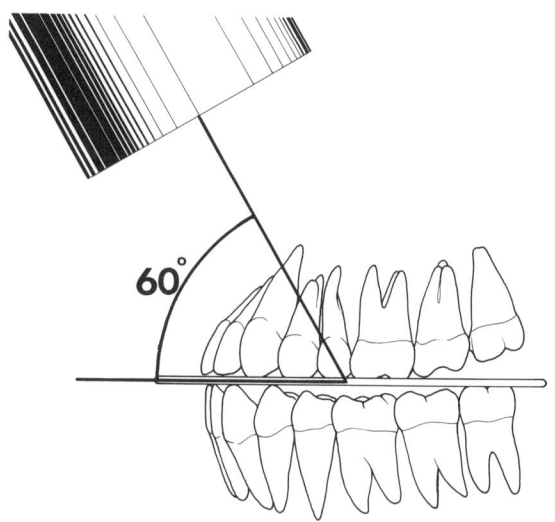

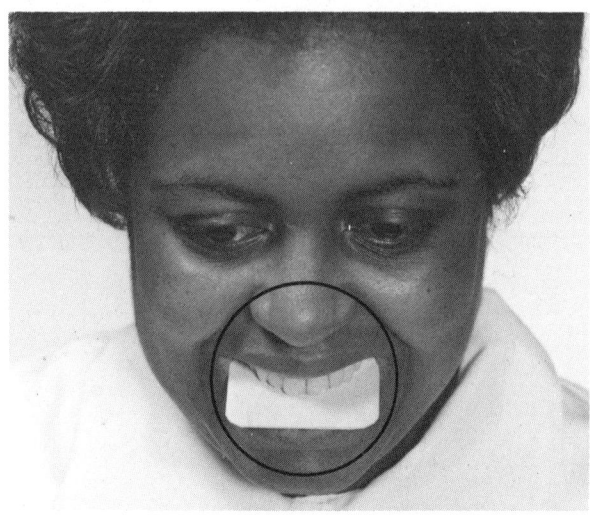

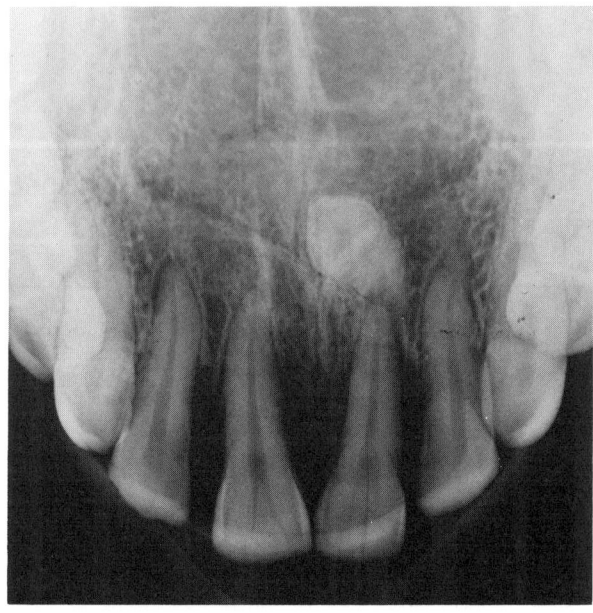

Fig. 12, V-6 Maxillary topographical occlusal projection.

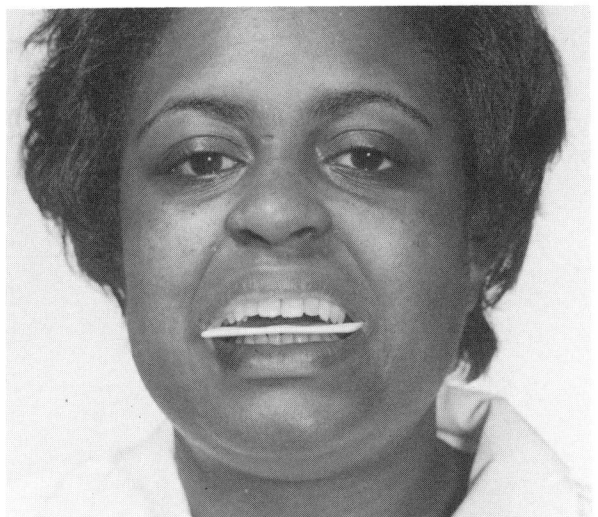

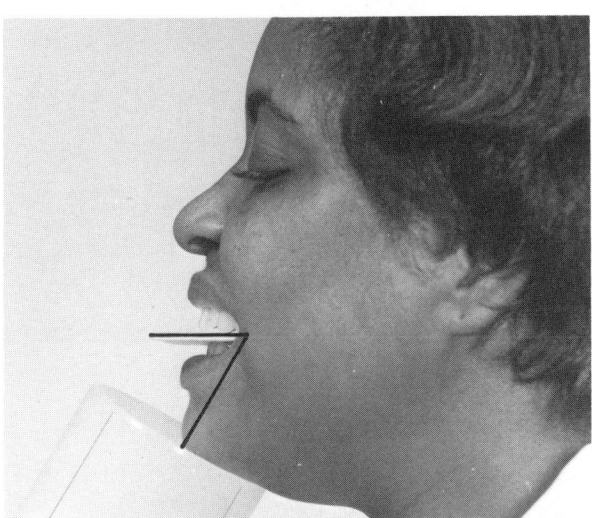

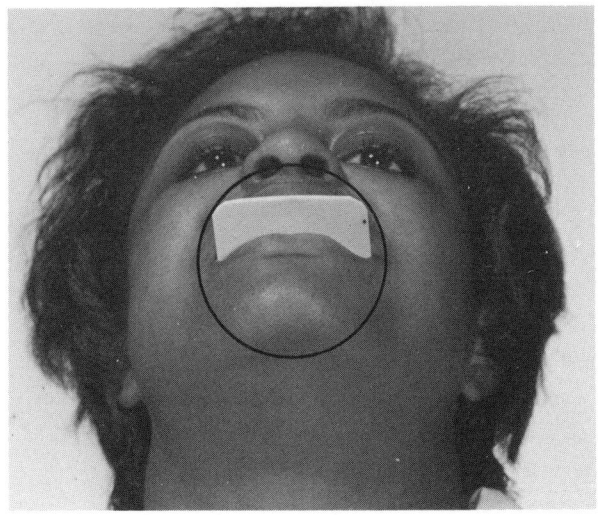

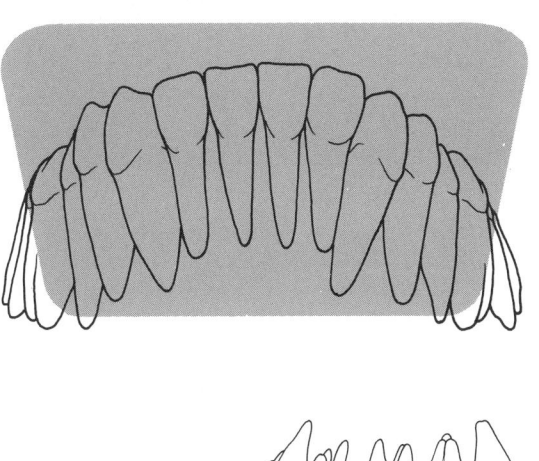

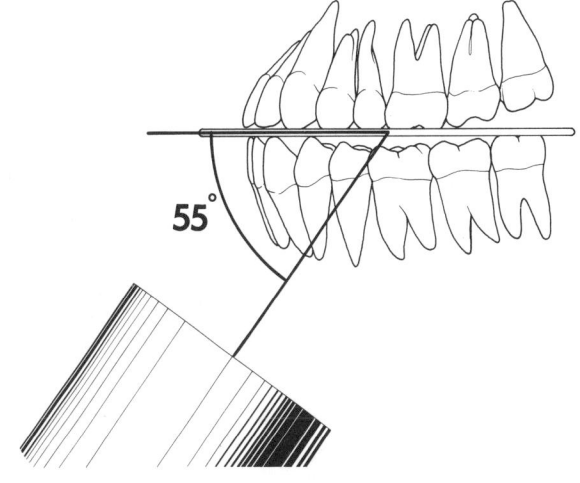

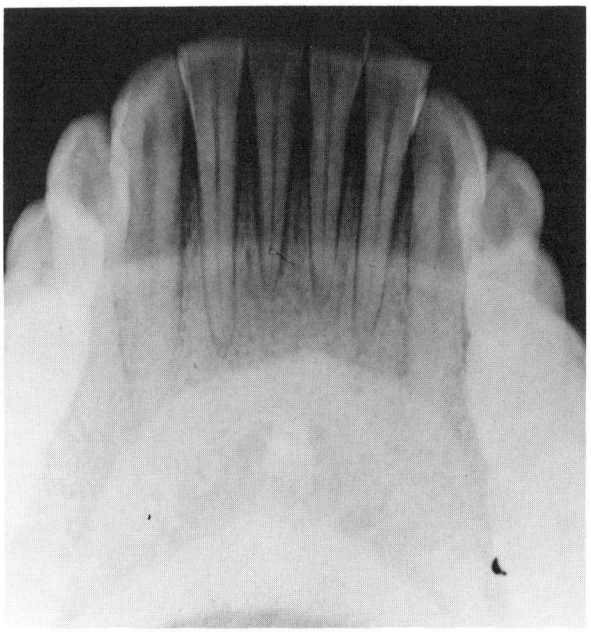

Fig. 13, V-6 Mandibular topographical occlusal projection.

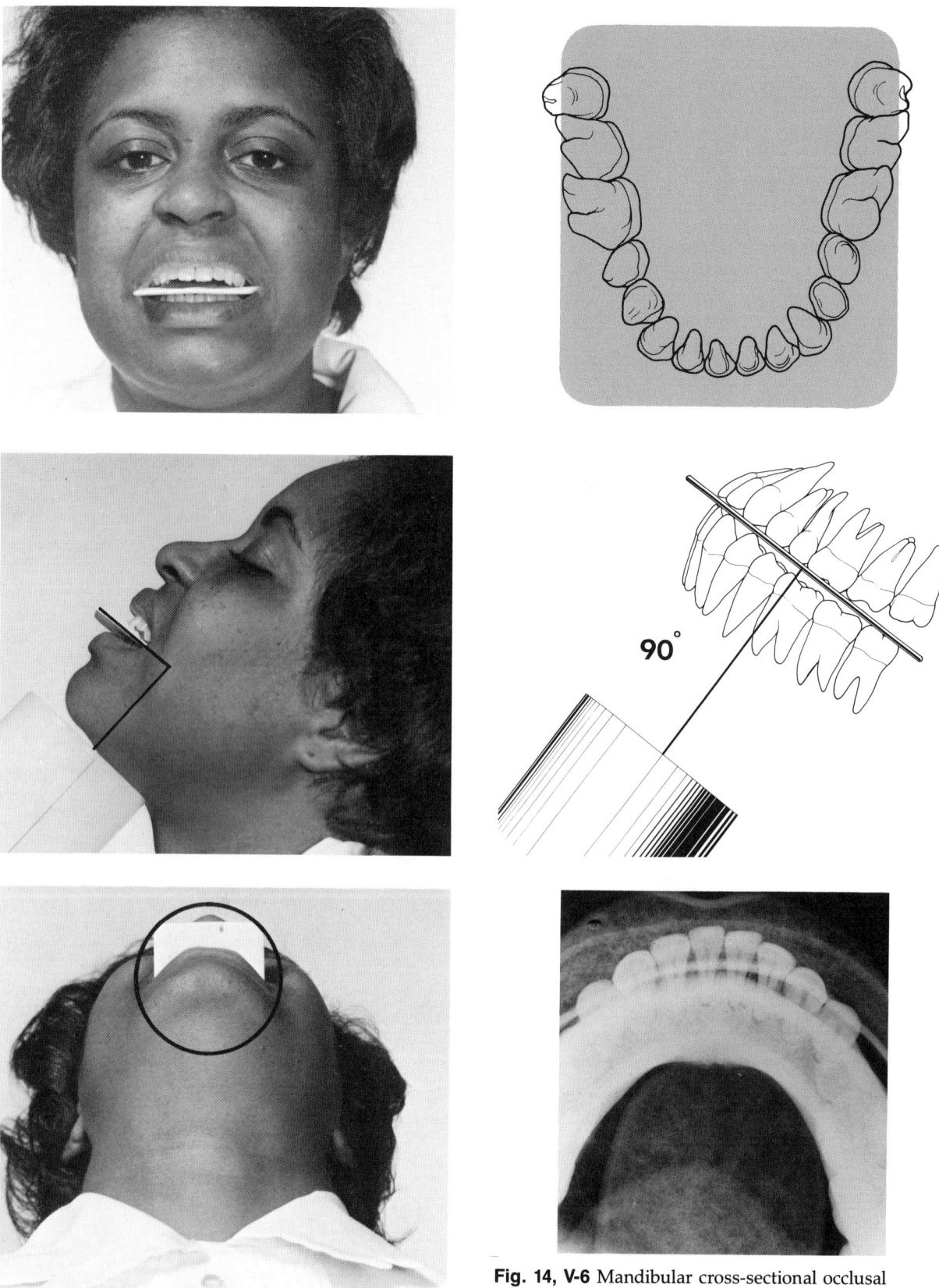

Fig. 14, V-6 Mandibular cross-sectional occlusal projection.

BIBLIOGRAPHY

Eastman Kodak Company. *X-Rays in Dentistry*. Rochester, N.Y.: Radiology Markets Division, 1985.

Frommer, H. H. *Radiology for Dental Auxiliaries*. 4th ed. St. Louis: C. V. Mosby Co., 1987.

Langland, O. E.; Langlais, R. P.; and Morris, C. R. *Principles and Practice of Panoramic Radiology*. Philadelphia: W. B. Saunders Co., 1982.

Langland, O. E.; Langlais, R. P.; Sippy, F. H.; and Williamson, G. *Radiology for Dental Hygienists and Dental Assistants*. Springfield, Ill.: Charles C. Thomas, 1988.

Section 6

Examination

In a few words, phrases, or sentences, answer the following questions. Use a separate sheet of paper.

1. What is the basic mechanism used to expose a panoramic radiograph?

2. List three indications for obtaining a panoramic film.

3. Give two reasons explaining why panoramic films show less image detail than periapical films.

4. List seven steps used in positioning a patient for a panorex radiograph.

5. Why are cephalometric films taken?

6. What is a cephalostat?

7. What are the indications for taking a lateral oblique mandible radiograph?

8. Describe the patient position and x-ray cone alignment used to obtain a lateral oblique mandibular projection.

9. What are the indications for taking radiographs of the temporomandibular joint?

10. Describe the patient position and x-ray cone alignment used to obtain a radiograph of the temporomandibular joint.

11. What are the indications for using the disto-oblique third molar technique?

12. What variations in cone alignment are used to take a third molar disto-oblique radiograph of the maxillary third molar?

13. What variations in cone alignment are used to take a third molar disto-oblique radiograph of a mandibular third molar?

14. Describe the packet placement and cone alignment used in obtaining a maxillary topographical radiograph.

15. Describe the packet placement and cone alignment used in obtaining a mandibular topographical radiograph.

Index